Healing with Spiritual Practices

Healing with Spiritual Practices

Proven Techniques for Disorders from Addictions and Anxiety to Cancer and Chronic Pain

Thomas G. Plante, PhD, ABPP, Editor

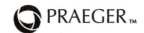

PRAEGER™

An Imprint of ABC-CLIO, LLC

Santa Barbara, California • Denver, Colorado

Library of Congress Cataloging-in-Publication Data

Names: Plante, Thomas G., editor.
Title: Healing with spiritual practices : proven techniques for disorders
   from addictions and anxiety to cancer and chronic pain / [edited by]
   Thomas G. Plante.
Description: Santa Barbara, California : Praeger, [2018] | Includes
   bibliographical references and index.
Identifiers: LCCN 2018010858 | ISBN 9781440860690 (print : alk. paper) |
   ISBN 9781440860706 (ebook)
Subjects: | MESH: Spiritual Therapies | Spirituality | Religion
Classification: LCC RZ401 | NLM WB 885 | DDC 615.8/52—dc23
LC record available at https://lccn.loc.gov/2018010858

ISBN: 978-1-4408-6069-0 (print)
     978-1-4408-6070-6 (ebook)

22 21 20 19 18   1 2 3 4 5

This book is also available as an eBook.

Praeger
An Imprint of ABC-CLIO, LLC

ABC-CLIO, LLC
130 Cremona Drive, P.O. Box 1911
Santa Barbara, California 93116-1911
www.abc-clio.com

This book is printed on acid-free paper ∞

Manufactured in the United States of America

*To my mother, Marcia Carol (McCormick) Plante,
who well modeled spiritual and religious coping through
faith, ritual, prayer, and, most especially, song,
and for all others who have used their talents in spiritual and
religious interventions and practices to help others
struggling with various challenges.*

Contents

Preface

There are few topics that receive as much attention, debate, and expression of strong emotion as religion. Many maintain that religious engagement is inspiration for great good in the world, such as remarkable examples of charity, love, kindness, and sacrifice. Yet others believe that religion provides the motivation for so much that is wrong with the world, such as hate, prejudice, intolerance, terrorism, and warfare. Perhaps a more reasonable, balanced, and evidence-based perspective would support the notion that religion and spirituality can bring out and inspire the very best and the very worst in people and that this has been true for centuries and even millennia. And certainly religious beliefs and practices have been used to help people and communities with a wide range of physical and mental health problems.

In recent years, quality academic research and scholarship has begun to investigate whether religious and spiritual practices and interventions can be effectively used in evidence-based health care using the very best methodological and statistical techniques available. These studies have sought to determine if religious and spiritual engagement can help people cope better or even help cure those who are ill from mental and physical health problems.

The purpose of this book is to bring together some of the best minds on this topic in order to offer thoughtful and evidence-based reflections about the potential benefits of religious and spiritual engagement in treating a wide range of health problems. Contributors come from multiple academic and clinical disciplines (e.g., psychology, nursing, medicine, occupational therapy), locations (e.g., United States, Canada, Israel), and religious traditions (e.g., Christian, Jewish, Buddhist). They also focus on diverse patient populations (e.g., children; elderly; and patients experiencing cancer, chronic pain, addictions, mental health challenges). This diversity provides a richness and multilayered approach to the book project. The topics and approaches presented are not exhaustive or encyclopedic but are more of a sampling and representation of areas where spiritual and religious engagement has been used effectively with research support to assist those who struggle with a variety of mental and physical health problems.

This book is a companion to several earlier edited books on this general topic published by Praeger/ABC-CLIO, including *The Psychology of Compassion and Cruelty: Understanding the Emotional, Spiritual, and Religious Influences of Religion* (2015), *Spirituality and Positive Psychology: Understanding the Psychological Fruits of Faith* (2012), *Contemplative Practices in Action: Spirituality, Meditation, and Health* (2010), and *Spirit, Science, and Health: How the Spiritual Mind Fuels Physical Wellness* (2007). Interested readers may wish to review them together.

Acknowledgments

So many people other than the author or editor help in the completion of a book project. Some contribute in a direct way, while others help out in a more supportive role. I would like to acknowledge the assistance of the many people who worked to make this book project a reality.

First and foremost, I would like to thank the contributors to this volume. They include some of the leading scholars and thinkers in the field and have been a stellar team to provide the reader with state-of-the-art and evidence-based reflection and scholarship. Second, it is important to recognize the wonderful people at ABC-CLIO who published this book. Most especially, many thanks to editor Debbie Carvalko for her efforts not only with this book project but also with other book projects that I have published with her assistance during the past few decades. Finally, I would like to thank my wife, Lori, and son, Zach, who are daily reminders that life is good and sacred and that I am blessed beyond words to have them both in my life.

CHAPTER ONE

Spiritually Formative Practices and Stress-Related Disorders

Everett L. Worthington Jr., Loren L. Toussaint,
Brandon J. Griffin, Don E. Davis, and
Joshua N. Hook

In this chapter, we propose that spiritually formative practices have the potential to alleviate stress-related health problems and promote well-being. Although this proposition has not been directly tested, we provide a theoretical rationale based on a psychological need to have a coherent sense of identity. People strive to be consistent. When people identify with a value but act inconsistently with that value, they experience dissonance. Dissonance may lead to anxiety, depression, anger, and negative health behaviors that exacerbate stress-related health problems. On the other hand, consistency between one's behavior and virtue-promoting values can lead to a sense of coherent identity that provides resources to cope with stress, enhancing outcomes such as subjective well-being, interpersonal connection, and religious/ spiritual well-being. As initial evidence pertinent to our theorizing, we explore associations between two virtuous practices—humility and forgiveness—and stress-related outcomes. We conclude that the rationale and evidence justify more scientific investigation of the impact of spiritually formative practices on stress-related disorders.

Definitions and Concepts

Spiritual formation has been practiced for millennia. Spiritually formative practices include any action or activity that one engages in with the intention of cultivating spirituality or spiritual experiences, including but not limited to meditation/prayer, reading sacred texts, receiving spiritual direction or instruction, and gathering as a community. Broadly speaking, *spirituality* is defined as closeness or intimacy with what one holds to be sacred. Davis and colleagues[1] describe sources of spiritualty that individuals often draw upon in their individual practices. Typically, religious spirituality involves expressing one's spirituality within a well-defined community of like-minded people sharing common beliefs, values, and practices (e.g., Buddhism, Christianity, Hinduism, Islam). Others might treat humanity as sacred, which would yield humanistic spirituality, or they might treat nature or the natural environment as sacred, which would yield nature spirituality. Still others seek to reach their own highest human potential, yielding self-spirituality, focusing inward for enlightenment. Finally, seeking the sacred outside of oneself or corporeal existence yields transcendent spirituality. Of course, any given individual can be moved by numerous types of spirituality.

Christian Spiritual Formation

As one example of spiritual formation, consider Christians who see spiritual formation as a process of being conformed to or having (more of) the mind of Christ. When Christians are converted (see Acts 9), they are born again (John 3:3) and become new creations (2 Cor. 5:17a); the old person is said to be dead, and the new person is enlivened by the Holy Spirit (2 Cor. 5:17b). They are enjoined to develop the mind of Christ (1 Cor. 2:16; Phil. 2:5), which is characterized first by humility (Rom. 12:3; Phil. 2:6–9). Romans 12:2 (all quotes are from the New International Version) says, "Do not conform to the pattern of this world, but be transformed by the renewing of your mind. Then you will be able to test and approve what God's will is—his good, pleasing and perfect will." In 2 Corinthians 3:18, Paul writes, "And we, who with unveiled faces all reflect the Lord's glory, are being transformed into his likeness with ever-increasing glory, which comes from the Lord, who is the Spirit." As Christians become transformed into more Christlike people, through the working of the Holy Spirit, the fruit of the Spirit—"love, joy, peace, forbearance, kindness, goodness, faithfulness, gentleness and self-control" (Gal. 5:22)—grows within them and is manifested outwardly.

Spiritual growth is not automatic. Rather, it requires both human effort and God's sovereign working. As Paul writes in his letter to the Ephesians (2:8–10), "For it is by grace you have been saved, through faith—and this is not from yourselves, it is the gift of God—not by works, so that no one can boast. For we are God's handiwork, created in Christ Jesus to do good works, which God prepared in advance for us to do." Nor is this considered to be solely human work. In Philippians 2:13, Paul writes, "For it is God who is at work in you, both to will and to work for his good pleasure." So Christian spiritual formation is a joint project by God's initiative and the Christian's responsiveness to form Christ's character within the believer, conforming the Christian to the template of Jesus's character. Furthermore, the project of building people into Christlikeness is also a community project, involving an unseen cloud of witnesses who have gone before (Heb. 12:1: "Therefore, since we are surrounded by such a great cloud of witnesses, let us throw off everything that hinders and the sin that so easily entangles. And let us run with perseverance the race marked out for us") and a community of believers who are contemporary with the Christian—parents, teachers, elders, exemplars, preachers, and fellow Christians who encourage each other, whether they are near or far from the Christian—all helping one another to move toward more Christlikeness (1 Thess. 5:11: "Therefore encourage one another and build each other up, just as in fact you are doing"; Rom. 14:19: "Let us therefore make every effort to do what leads to peace and to mutual edification [i.e., upbuilding].").

Methods of Christian Spiritual Formation

Over the centuries, many of the methods by which Christians form each other in line with the work of the Holy Spirit have become institutions. People start their journey toward Christlikeness by taking encouragement to begin from scripture or their local religious leaders. Then they engage in systematic spiritual practices. These started with the early church members encouraging one another. As the author of Hebrews writes, "And let us consider how we may spur one another on toward love and good deeds, not giving up meeting together, as some are in the habit of doing, but encouraging one another—and all the more as you see the Day approaching" (Heb. 10:24–25). The practices progressed to those initiated by the desert forbears,[2] who practiced piety in the wilderness, and later to people who withdrew into convents and orders in the church and practiced spiritual disciplines within a close community of people who were struggling with the same spiritual growth issues and temptations and could admonish, teach, and encourage each other. These include things like listening to sermons that teach, admonish, and encourage; heeding prophets who speak God's truth to people; attending Christian education programs in churches, seminaries, universities, or high schools; practicing spiritual disciplines (e.g., prayer, silence, solitude, fasting); taking spiritual direction; listening to or watching Christian speakers, teachers, radio stations, television programming, podcasts, and YouTube clips; watching Christian drama; reading Christian novels; and all manner of teaching and training methods adapted from secular and church-based methods to help people grow in closeness to God and in fellowship with Jesus, the Holy Spirit, and the Christian community, even in the face of temptations and suffering. These efforts to behave virtuously extend to the ways people treat others who do not name Christ as their lord and to reshape the world into a socially just realm.

Thus, Christian virtue formation worked through three steps to yield spiritual satisfaction. Usually, the emphasis of efforts to help promote spiritual formation involved first having a goal of becoming more Christlike. The idea was to conform behavior and attitude to approximate Christ's. That was understood to involve simultaneously complete reliance on the Holy Spirit and effortful practice in learning, acting, and seeking to develop Christlike attitudes. It was understood that one must respond well under testing, so some spiritual formation methods built in rigorous self-control tests and confession, repentance, and absolution rituals for inevitable failures. Some methods entailed tests like fasting. Others expected that rigorous duties and schedules for prayer, devotion, scripture reading, and meditation would be their own tests. When life tested people through suffering (e.g., illness, losses), people were expected to cope faithfully. In short, spiritual formation was based on a virtue-building paradigm, and although there are many ways to form Christian character, we will focus on virtue development.

Christians, and other spiritual people, often use worldly ways to build spiritual closeness. This is analogous to building a concrete structure by using a wooden frame (i.e., ways of the physical world) and asking God to fill the frame with inner concrete (i.e., character development in a way that gets the person closer to God) to form the weight-bearing walls, columns, or other structures that will hold up the edifice of a Christian character and allow a Christian community to benefit.

Classic Virtue Theory

The Christian method of virtue formation paralleled those developed in secular societies. A summary of a classic virtue-building model involves four steps.[3] First, the person sees the goal. The sight is more a glimpse than a clear-sighted focus because people cannot precisely anticipate what the virtue might look like in their lives when it is fully formed. Second, the person practices the virtuous beliefs, values, and acts until the particular virtue becomes a habit of the heart or tacit knowledge (as opposed to focal knowledge[4]). Third, the person undergoes numerous self-imposed or life-imposed tests, trials, temptations, and suffering. All of those, one hopes, can strengthen the virtue. One way this strengthening occurs is through tests, trials, temptations, and suffering that may temporarily erode the virtue but allow a person the opportunity to become aware of and respond to limitations, which serves to increase the robustness of the virtue across contexts. Fourth, the person gains a sense of ultimate satisfaction from the practice of the virtue.

What Are Christian Virtues?

Virtue is excellence in doing right acts. Vices are spiritually and morally harmful acts. The Christian church developed within a culturally Greek world. Historically, four Greek virtues were adopted by the church: justice, self-control, courage, and prudent wisdom. The church added three distinctive Christian virtues from the writing of Paul in 1 Corinthians 13 (i.e., faith, hope, and love). As the community of Christians developed, other Christian virtues were included. We might think of these as virtues emergent from close community interactions. They included forgiveness, humility, mutual submission, respect for authority, freedom with responsibility, social justice, loyalty, faithfulness, gratitude, hospitality, and generosity. The virtues practiced in Christian communities apparently differed from those practiced in secular Greek culture. They differed in telos (or end goal) of the virtue, methods by which virtues were thought to become habits of the heart, specific character traits that were considered virtuous, the priority ordering of the virtues, the outworking of virtues into daily life, and whether virtue or something else was the central goal of life itself.

The Seven Deadly Sins

Vices were to be eschewed as being antithetical to one who has the mind of Christ. Over time, as Schimmel[5] has argued, the vices became increasingly often summarized as seven deadly sins: pride, greed, lust, envy, gluttony, wrath, and sloth. Among psychological accounts, Schimmel[5] has argued that people are engaged in a personal, ongoing battle with sin and vice. The deadly sins have become iconic opponents people struggle against, and personal unhappiness and lack of fulfillment are products of giving in to their practice. Schimmel[5] uses philosophical, religious, and cultural accounts to draw lessons about how avoiding sin and practicing virtue can result in more fulfillment and health.

From Where Do Virtues Come?

Virtue and vice spring from the character, which, for religious and spiritual people, is built up over time through spiritual formation. That formation can be built in from parenting, community, reading, belonging to a virtue-seeking community, or a relationship with God involving listening and heeding direct communication from God and wise people. So virtues spring from within, but having said that, we admit that it is not that simple. If it were, the virtuous person would always be virtuous.

Rather, psychology tells us that situations are powerful. They provide external cues that trigger behavior directly, trigger internal cues (i.e., thoughts, feelings, memories, associations, reflexes, intuitions) that become salient and guide behavior, and trigger internal sequences of practiced behaviors (i.e., habits) that are engaged in almost automatically. People might value virtues, but situations can temporarily dominate behavior, subduing internal values in a particular situation. Furthermore, humans have many self-serving biases and heuristics of which they are unaware, and those biases and heuristics can short-circuit usual valued virtues.

Virtue-Vice Dissonance

Religious people try to build character virtues and reduce vices. There is not a one-to-one correspondence, but usually practicing vices puts us out of sorts with the Divine, community, close relationships, and our own psychological integrity. Typically, religious people's goal is to act consistently with deeply held valued virtues and not succumb to temptations to engage in vices. Psychologically, this is a human desire. Humans usually strive to be consistent.

According to social identity theory,[6] people identify with salient social groups (and with the people within them). They categorize and identify themselves with groups that establish their self-images.[6] Individuals remain in groups that share their values and are beneficial to them. Religious communities are formed and operate upon shared values. In Christianity, fellow believing Christians are seen as being adopted into a common family by God (Rom. 8:15). Thus, Christian identity, as in other religious groups, is partially rooted in communities of fellow believers—as well as with identification with God through Jesus.

In fact, people have numerous social identities that are defined by the different social groups with which they identify. Having several social identities relates to health because this gives people a larger social-support network to cope with stress.[7,8] But Christians whose identities are rooted within the congregations to which they belong—and perhaps other groups that overlap with people in their Christian congregations—still endure interpersonal transgressions within their own congregation. People stay in organizations and social groups that agree with their self-concept. They seek to align their inner virtues and their outward situations that trigger consonant virtues. This is because all people have various social identities that organize their inner and outer lives.[6,7] For some people, social identity is strong and consistent. For others, social identity is less well formed and organized and is inconsistent. To the extent that group membership provides a sense of social identity, people who are active in groups experience a positive effect on their physical and mental health, known as a "social cure."[7] Most people desire a consistent social identity, and when they act in opposition to that identity, they experience a sense of inconsistency, lack of balance,[9] and dissonance.

Cognitive dissonance theory originated by Festinger and Alto[10] suggested that people want to be self-consistent. That drive is so strong that people will change their beliefs and behaviors to maintain a sense of consistency. When identity is threatened, people experience stress. Stress motivates coping attempts to return to homeostasis or allostasis.[11] When people are stressed, they desire to relieve the stress through coping behaviors. Thus, dissonance can result in stress reactions, some of which may be profound and long-lasting, exacerbating stress-related physical, psychological, relational, and spiritual problems. Achieving consistency between one's values and behaviors through engaging in spiritually formative practices may be one way that individuals might meaningfully interpret and work to resolve dissonance.

Virtue-Vice Dissonance and Stress-Related Health Problems

What are the consequences of maintaining an incoherent sense of self by engaging in value-incongruent behavior rather than spiritually formative practice? We propose that this inconsistency has both biopsychosocial and spiritual consequences.

Biopsychosocial Effects

There are several dissonance-related biopsychosocial effects. Cortisol is a neurohormone intended to prepare bodily systems to deal with acute stressors. It often works in conjunction with adrenaline (i.e., epinephrine), and the balance of the two, or imbalance, can lead to stress-related disorders.[11] Sapolsky[12] investigated the physical effects of persistently high levels of cortisol. Chronically high levels of cortisol atrophy portions of the brain (often drastically) like the hippocampus, which consolidates memories, place people at risk for cardiovascular problems, dysregulate the sinus rhythms and make the parasympathetic nervous system malfunction with low heart rate variability, negatively affect the digestive system, dysregulate the immune system, affect the respiratory system, and cause malfunctions in the sexual and reproductive systems.

People might cope with the stress of identity inconsistency by changing health-related behaviors. For example, they might increase their drinking; self-medicate with pharmaceuticals (legal or otherwise); withdraw from social interaction and community (with attendant loss of social support); and not take care of themselves physically, mentally, relationally, or spiritually.

They also might cease or reduce physical activity due to feelings of increased stress. They might seek solace in smoking or other addictive behaviors, like gambling. They might feel a loss of self-esteem, and with the feelings of internal negativity, they might seek to create an external bodily reality that reflects the poor inward state they feel—engaging in behaviors like anorexia, cutting, or self-harm. On top of this, they might feel guilty and ashamed that they are not coping well, and self-condemnation might lead to negative outcomes on top of other outcomes.

Spiritual Effects

Wuthnow[13] suggests that most people spend the majority of their lives in a state of spiritual dwelling, which is a relatively stable state of relationship with what one considers sacred. However, when inconsistencies arise with their spiritual worldview or congruence with the social aspect of a faith community and their beliefs, practices, or values are called into question, people seek to resolve the inconsistency. That results in a time of seeking. Seeking is usually more stressful relative to dwelling; however, sometimes people can become comfortable with seeking. Williamson and Sandage[14] has investigated this tendency to spiritually dwell or seek. They have examined seminary students who often face challenging beliefs and practices relative to what they experienced prior to seminary. When seeking, people can become unmoored from the familiar and stable. They can feel alienated from God (or whatever they call sacred), close relationships, family, and community.

When people who value virtue find themselves unable or unwilling to act virtuously, they might feel a sense of inconsistency. People need a coherent sense of self. Thus, the threat of inconsistency creates stress. If the inconsistency is not rectified quickly, it can lead to anxiety, depression, anger, and health behaviors that promote illness, not good health. On the other hand, consistency with virtue-promoting values can lead to calm, tranquility, and peace—for example, if a committed Christian acts virtuously in forgiving; manifesting humility; and being patient, loving, compassionate, self-controlled, sympathetic, and empathic. Those positive feelings promote a broaden-and-build perspective[15] and lead to well-being.

Spiritually formative practices tend to be prosocial. Thus, they are reinforced in relationships, groups, communities, and society. Social reinforcement of such virtuous behavior also reaffirms one's desire to act virtuously and, when one is engaging in vice, heightens the sense of inconsistency and stress.

If consistency is important, we might ask what might happen if a person was, by character, vicious. If a vicious person acted consistently with his or her vices, should we expect the person to experience health and well-being? No. Consistency with vice-promoting values does not lead to the same physical and mental health and relational and spiritual outcomes as does consistency with virtue-promoting values because society's values are acting in opposition to the vicious person's personal values. Society generally punishes behaviors that are consistent with vice. Thus, practicing virtues, by a person who values virtue, brings correspondence, consistency, peace, and relief from stress, as well as better physical, mental, and relational health along with better spiritual health in the long run.

Spiritual Formation through Forgiveness and Humility

Virtues that govern the strengthening and repair of social bonds, such as forgiveness and humility, provide a key starting place for evaluating our theorizing on the role of spiritual formation. For both virtues, substantial basic research has set the stage for conducting interventions designed to promote habits that increasingly instill these virtues into relationships with other people of faith. Forgiveness and humility are also virtues that involve persistent challenges to maintaining healthy relationships.

The consistent practice of forgiveness indicates a commitment to one's social bonds within a community, even when hurts or disagreements threaten to damage those social bonds. Allowing resentment and rumination to go unchecked not only increases personal stress but creates a context in which retaliation and gossip can fester. Especially for valued relationships, forgiveness is a strong investment in giving a relationship an opportunity to grow stronger after offenses because it arrests the escalation of negative thoughts, feelings, and behaviors.

Similarly, humility involves the regulation of egotism or the demands one places on relationships. Humble people both generate margin and then share that surplus within valued relationships. The regular practice of becoming a person who seeks to contribute more than one consumes (i.e., a "big ego" sucks up all the air in the room, takes too much credit, feels entitled to more than others, etc.) is a discipline that can lead to a steady strengthening and stabilization of one's network of social bonds, which helps reinforce the development of character and has been linked to a variety of stress-related benefits. Prior interventions to promote these two virtues have relied on time-limited programs, but it may make sense to think of ways to pair these interventions with participants' existing spiritual formative practices in order to encourage longer-term habits designed to reinforce virtues pertaining to curbing retaliation or hoarding of scarce resources.

Forgiveness

The research on enhancing forgiveness through spiritually formative practice has developed in recent years.[16-19] For example, Vasiliauskas and McMinn[20] conducted an intervention study that explored the potential benefits of prayer among Christians who sought to forgive an interpersonal offense. Participants were 411 undergraduate students at private Christian colleges. They were randomly assigned to a prayer condition, a devotional attention condition, or a no-contact control condition. People in the prayer condition engaged in a 16-day devotional reading and prayer intervention focused on forgiveness. Those in the devotional attention condition meditated on devotional readings not related to forgiveness. People in both prayer and devotional attention conditions forgave more, but those in the prayer intervention condition also experienced more empathy toward their offender.

Greer and colleagues[16] adapted for Christians a workbook version of REACH Forgiveness, which was created for secular populations.[21,22] In benchmarking analyses, they compared the results of the workbook to three group interventions of nominally six hours in length. The mean d for these six-hour group studies was 0.61. For Greer and colleagues,[16] the pooled d across four forgiveness measures was $d = 1.37$.

Although no study has examined whether the spiritually formative pursuit of forgiveness has benefits to physical and mental health, we can adduce strong evidence that increasing forgiveness would result in improvements to mental and physical health. Wade and colleagues[23] did an extensive meta-analysis of randomized controlled studies of forgiveness interventions. Of forgiveness intervention trials, 10 assessed depression as an outcome and 7 assessed anxiety. The d for reducing depression was $d = 0.34$ and for reducing anxiety was $d = 0.63$.

These intervention studies did not assess physical stress-related variables, so any conclusions about their efficacy to treat stress-related physical disorders is speculative based on extrapolating from mental health variables. Waltman and colleagues[24] have used Enright and Fitzgibbons's[25] process model to intervene on anger-recall stress-induced changes in myocardial perfusion and forgiveness. Patients ($N = 32$) were administered a baseline and anger-recall stress-imaging protocol. Of the participants, 17 who demonstrated anger-recall stress-induced myocardial perfusion defects were randomly assigned to 10 weekly interpersonal forgiveness ($n = 9$) or control ($n = 8$) therapy sessions. After treatment, they did the test again at posttest and at a 10-week follow-up. Patients who did the forgiveness intervention had fewer anger-recall stress-induced myocardial perfusion defects.

Humility

Humility is at the heart of spiritual formation as it is conceptualized by many belief systems. However, the psychological study of interventions to promote humility is in its infancy.

Research on humility has accumulated rapidly recently; however, intervention research is much less developed, although initial results are promising. Two full-fledged workbook intervention studies have been conducted. Lavelock and colleagues[22] had people complete a nine-hour workbook and compared them to a control condition. They assessed the degree to which completing the humility intervention built humility and other virtues, specifically forgiveness, patience, and self-control. They also assessed positivity in terms of increased positive emotions and decreased negative emotions. The PROVE Humility workbook produced an increase in humility (d = 0.47), forgiveness (d = 0.56), patience (d = 0.49), and self-control (d = 0.10) relative to the control condition. Lavelock and colleagues[22] replicated this with a revised version of the workbook. The humility workbook produced increases in humility (d = 0.86), forgiveness (d = 0.91), and patience (d = 0.19).

Future Research on Spiritual Formation and Stress-Related Disorders

Currently, there is only indirect evidence from psychological studies that spiritual formation exercises can reduce the level of stress-related disorders or prevent them altogether, make people resilient when they occur, or promote states in which such disorders are resisted. However, there is theoretical reason to believe that such effects are possible. This leaves a research agenda wide open. In general, basic research should focus on testing whether the theoretical reasoning linking spiritual formation as an antagonist to stress-related disorders is sound. This might address such propositions as the assumption that spiritual formation results in less chronic stress, and if so, for whom and under what conditions. The idea that unforgiveness, lack of humility, impatience, lack of gratitude, lack of generosity, and the opposites of each of the panoply of virtues are stressful might be a very tenuous assumption indeed. For example, as Chester and DeWall[26] have shown, for some people, revenge is sweet. We might also think that miserliness (instead of generosity) might settle some people because they hoard their resources and thus feel more secure. One could speculate as well about all the other virtues.

In terms of intervention research, developing targeted virtue-oriented interventions that can be used in spiritual formation is a must for all religions and spiritual worldviews for each of the constituent virtues and assessing as an outcome whether they yield lessened stress-related disorders, prevention, resilience, or promotion of resistance to stress. The assumption that becoming more virtuous in more virtues develops one's spiritual formation and reduces the impact of stress-related disorders deserves testing.

Most of the existing research in this area has focused on college students. Future research is also needed in religious communities of various sizes. It is conceivable that megachurches are highly different environments for developing oneself spiritually than are small local congregations. While the large congregations have more resources and more money for programming, the social connections might not be as tight, and social groups might be where spiritual formation is most effective. For the researcher who studies virtues within religious contexts, this research area is one that a career could be built around, with connections both to positive psychology and to religious groups.

References

1. Davis, D. E., Rice, K., Hook, J. N., Van Tongeren, D. R., DeBlaere, C., Choe, E., & Worthington, E. L. (2015). Development of the Sources of Spirituality Scale. *Journal of Counseling Psychology, 62*(3), 503–513.

2. Merton, T. (1970). *Wisdom of the desert.* New York: New Directions Publishing.

3. Worthington, E. L. Jr., Lavelock, C., Van Tongeren, D. R., Jennings, D. J., Gartner, A. L., Davis, D. E., & Hook, J. N. (2014). Virtue in positive psychology. In K. Timpe & C. Boyd (Eds.), *Virtues and their vices* (pp. 433–457). New York: Oxford University Press.

4. Polanyi, M. (1967). *The tacit dimension.* Garden City, NY: Doubleday Anchor Books.

5. Schimmel, S. (1997). *The seven deadly sins: Jewish, Christian, and classical reflections on human nature.* Oxford, England: Oxford University Press.

6. Tajfel, H., & Turner, J. C. (1986). The social identity theory of intergroup behavior. In S. Worchel & W. G. Austin (Eds.), *Psychology of intergroup relations* (pp. 7–24). Chicago, IL: Nelson-Hall.

7. Jetten, J., Haslam, S. A., Cruwys, T., Greenaway, K. H., Haslam, C., & Steffens, N. K. (2017). Advancing the social identity approach to health and well-being: Progressing the social cure research agenda. *European Journal of Social Psychology, 47*(7), 789–802.

8. Steffens, N. K., Haslam, S. A., Schuh, S. C., Jetten, J., & van Dick, R. (2017). A meta-analytic review of social identification and health in organizational contexts. *Personality and Social Psychology Review, 21*(4), 303–335.

9. Heider, F. (1958). *The psychology of interpersonal relations.* New York: Wiley.

10. Festinger, L., & Alto, C. A. (1957). *A theory of cognitive dissonance.* Palo Alto, CA: Stanford University Press.

11. McEwen, B. S., & Lasley, E. N. (2002). *The end of stress as we know it.* New York: Dana Press.

12. Sapolsky, R. M. (2004). *Why zebras don't get ulcers* (3rd ed.). New York: Henry Holt Publishers.

13. Wuthnow, R. (1998). *After heaven: Spirituality in America since the 1950s.* Berkeley, CA: University of California Press.

14. Williamson, I. T., & Sandage, S. J. (2009). Longitudinal analyses of religious and spiritual development among seminary students. *Mental Health, Religion & Culture, 12*(8), 787–801.

15. Fredrickson, B. L. (2001). The role of positive emotions in positive psychology: The broaden-and-build theory of positive emotions. *The American Psychologist, 56*(3), 218–226.

16. Greer, C. L., Worthington, E. L., Jr., Lin, Y., Lavelock, C. R., & Griffin, B. J. (2014). Efficacy of a self-directed forgiveness workbook for Christian victims of within-congregation offenders. *Spirituality in Clinical Practice, 1*(3), 218–230.

17. Lampton, C., Oliver, G., Worthington, E. L., Jr., & Berry, J. W. (2005). Helping Christian college students become more forgiving: An intervention study to promote forgiveness as part of a program to shape Christian character. *Journal of Psychology and Theology, 33,* 278–290.

18. Stratton, S. P., Dean, J. B., Nooneman, A. J., Bode, R. A., & Worthington, E. L., Jr. (2008). Forgiveness interventions as spiritual development strategies: Workshop training, expressive writing about forgiveness, and retested controls. *Journal of Psychology and Christianity, 27,* 347–357.

19. Worthington, E. L., Jr., Hunter, J. L., Sharp, C. B., Hook, J. N., Van Tongeren, D. R., Davis, D. E., . . . Monforte-Milton, M. M. (2010). A psychoeducational intervention to promote forgiveness in Christians in the Philippines. *Journal of Mental Health Counseling, 32*(1), 82–103.

20. Vasiliauskas, S. L., & McMinn, M. R. (2013). The effects of a prayer intervention on the process of forgiveness. *Psychology of Religion and Spirituality, 5*(1), 23–32.

21. Harper, Q., Worthington, E. L., Griffin, B. J., Lavelock, C. R., Hook, J. N., Vrana, S. R., & Greer, C. L. (2014). Efficacy of a workbook to promote forgiveness: A randomized controlled trial with university students. *Journal of Clinical Psychology, 70*(12), 1158–1169.

22. Lavelock, C. R., Worthington, E. L., Jr., Griffin, B. J., Garthe, R. C., Elnasseh, A., Davis, D. E., & Hook, J. N. (2017). Still waters run deep: Humility as a master virtue. *Journal of Psychology and Theology, 45*(4), 286–303.

23. Wade, N. G., Cornish, M. A., Tucker, J. R., Worthington, E. L., Jr., Sandage, S., & Rye, M. (in press). Promoting forgiveness: Characteristics of the treatment, the clients, and their interaction. *Journal of Counseling Psychology.*

24. Waltman, M. A., Russell, D. C., Coyle, C. T., Enright, R. D., Holter, A. C., & Swoboda, C. M. (2009). The effects of a forgiveness intervention on patients with coronary artery disease. *Psychology & Health, 24*(1), 11–27.

25. Enright, R. D., Fitzgibbons, R. P., & Washington, D. C. (2014). *Forgiveness therapy: An empirical guide for resolving anger and restoring hope.* Washington, DC: American Psychological Association.

26. Chester, D. S., & DeWall, C. N. (2016). The pleasure of revenge: Retaliatory aggression arises from a neural imbalance toward reward. *Social Cognitive and Affective Neuroscience, 11*(7), 1173–1182.

CHAPTER TWO

Nurturing Hope: Tools for Cultivating Hopeful Thinking and a Meaningful Life

David B. Feldman and Sophie von Garnier

Hope has engaged the human imagination as long as we have had stories to pass from generation to generation. One of the earliest accounts of hope can be found in Hesiod's (750–650 BCE) myth of Pandora.[1] The first human woman, the beautiful Pandora, was given a strange box by the gods. Despite being warned not to open it, Pandora couldn't resist. And, in that moment, "all the miseries that spell sorrow for men" (p. 164) escaped the vessel, explaining the existence of pain and suffering in the world.[1] According to the legend, however, after Pandora slammed the lid closed again, one thing remained inside: hope. To this day, humankind continues to hold on to hope as an asset that aids in perseverance even through its darkest hours.

In addition to its role in ancient Greek mythology, hope has been present in many religious faiths but in different forms. In Christianity, for instance, believers' hopes are placed in the return of Jesus Christ, who the faithful believe will bring about the final judgment and resurrection of his followers. The ultimate hope is for one's immortal soul to be with God for eternity. According to Ogden, "God's love . . . therefore is itself not only the *why* of Christian hope but also its *for what* [emphases added]" (p. 159).[2]

Buddhism's path to enlightenment is more concerned with truly being in the present moment as opposed to placing hope in desired future events. Given the Buddhist belief that all earthly things are impermanent and subject to change, it is problematic to pin one's hope on any of them.[3] Unlike in the Western tradition, hopelessness is embraced for its ability to free the individual. As Pema Chödrön has written, "by giving up all hope of alternatives to the present moment" (p. 45), people are able to lead more joyful lives.[4] Yet Buddhism does not fully close the door on experiencing hope in a way that Westerners might more easily relate to. Buddhist scholar Josei Toda explained that the most persevering people do not place their hopes on personal desires but, instead, base them on their deep wish for the happiness of every human being on earth, thereby remaining undefeated by life's often tremendous hardships.[5]

Despite hope's role in many spiritual and religious traditions, it was not until recently that it was accepted as a subject worthy of empirical study. In 1959, the influential psychiatrist Karl Menninger not only recognized its value, placing hope alongside "its immortal sisters, Faith and Love," but also implored his colleagues, "are we not now duty bound to speak up as scientists, not about a new rocket . . . but about this ancient but rediscovered truth, the validity of Hope in human development [?]" (p. 491).[6]

Given its rich history, there are countless ways to understand hope. It is the psychologist's very unromantic job to pin down complex constructs like hope, rendering them scientifically testable and useful as mental-health tools. In this spirit, the definition of hope used throughout this chapter is based on C. R. Snyder's hope theory, the most widely used model of the phenomenon in the psychological literature. While his conceptualization may not serve to inspire mythological narratives, it explains the practical mechanisms through which hope affects long-term well-being and thus provides a foothold for nurturing this important asset in day-to-day life.[7,8]

Perhaps most notably, hope theory shows that it's possible to be hopeful even when things aren't going our way. That's because hope is a future-focused phenomenon. That is, hope primarily involves the *belief that the future can be better*. As such, we can be unhappy with the way things are presently going in our lives yet remain hopeful that our actions today could make a difference tomorrow.

According to Snyder, hope thrives when three basic conditions are met in our lives. The first condition is having a goal: something for which to hope. Goals can be anything that we desire to get, do, be, experience, or create.[7] They can vary from quite small, taking only a few minutes to achieve (e.g., dropping off one's children at school on time), to extremely large, requiring many years to accomplish (e.g., saving for their college education). They can be in any area of life, ranging from career objectives, like meeting monthly sales quotas and climbing corporate ladders, to social and even spiritual goals, like being a more loving partner or a more faithful Christian, Jew, Muslim, Hindu, or Buddhist. Whatever the specifics, the key to most effectively setting this first condition for hope to thrive is to adopt goals that are personally meaningful, that provide a sense of purpose.

The second condition for hope to thrive involves our ability to plot pathways. A pathway is a strategy or plan for achieving a goal. While pathways can be simple or complex, the important thing for nurturing hope is to choose to do *something* that will positively contribute (even in a small way) to achieving whatever goal we have embraced. Goals are rarely achieved all at once but rather one step at a time. Of course, life often throws curve balls, and at least some of our pathways will eventually become blocked. For this reason, hopeful people often produce multiple pathways in order to circumvent possible obstacles to reaching a goal.

The third and final condition for hope to thrive involves nurturing personal agency. *Agency* refers to the motivation or sense of empowerment that pushes us to strive for our goals. Agency derives primarily from positive beliefs about ourselves and our capabilities. As in Watty Piper's children's book, *The Little Engine That Could*, high-agency beliefs, such as "I think I can," fuel our hope and motivate us to act.[9]

Snyder argued that hope is shaped by our learning history. As children, we all were confronted with challenging experiences that taught us the degree to which our efforts affect our ability to achieve desired outcomes.[8] With repeated learning experiences throughout the life span, whether successes or failures, we develop our personal senses of agency and pathways.[8]

Although goals, pathways, and agency are distinct conditions that can be set somewhat independently of one another in our lives, they constantly influence each other. If we begin pursuing a goal with high agency but cannot develop effective pathways, our initially upbeat agency thoughts (e.g., "I am capable of accomplishing this goal") will soon sour as our hope begins to stagnate (e.g., "Maybe I can't do this"). Likewise, if we have generated numerous pathways to a goal but are unable to conjure sufficient agency, we will likely begin rejecting many of these pathways, believing they are not workable. Finally, if no goals exist at all, there is no opportunity for pathways and agency to develop in the first place. Thus, hope cannot fully exist unless all three of these conditions are present.

The three conditions for hope to thrive are essential in many areas of life. Consider the example of pursuing a college degree. Students begin by clearly formulating this intention (i.e., setting their *goal*). They then may pursue various *pathways* to maximize their chances of success—taking an ACT study course, seeking a writing tutor to help them with their application essay, or applying to multiple schools. Finally, they must conjure sufficient *agency* to persistently pursue these pathways, perhaps by reminding themselves of their past successes, personal strengths, or the meaningfulness of their aspirations.

But hope is not limited to practical goals. Spiritual goals also require the three conditions for hope to thrive. If practicing Christians, for instance, desire to foster the virtue of forgiveness in themselves, they first must clearly set this intention (i.e., goal). Their religious tradition may then offer various pathways to help them along their journey, perhaps including reading religious literature, praying for personal change, or speaking with a pastor. In order to do this, they may use the strength of their faith as motivation (i.e., agency).

What Are the Benefits of Hope?

Hope (as defined above) is related to a variety of positive outcomes across different life domains. According to research, high-hope individuals experience more frequent positive emotions, have a greater sense of meaning in life, feel more satisfied with their lives, and experience greater self-esteem than their low-hope counterparts.[10–13] Moreover, they more often follow through on their intentions and, when faced with obstacles standing in the way of their goals, are better at circumnavigating them.[14,15] When life stressors inevitably occur, hopeful individuals also use healthier coping mechanisms.[16] Perhaps for this reason, higher hope is related to lower levels of depression, anxiety, and suicidal ideation.[10,11,17]

In terms of personal success, multiple studies have shown that hope predicts not only academic achievement but also college retention and timely graduation.[18–21] In both children and young adults, higher hope levels are related to higher test scores and higher GPAs.[22–25] Hope also has been shown to work as a buffer against stressful life events in middle and high school students, leading to higher life satisfaction.[26] Finally, Hirschi found that hopeful adults were more likely to engage in proactive career behaviors, such as networking.[27]

Hope also benefits families who are dealing with stressful situations. Kashdan and colleagues found that higher-hope parents adapted more easily than their lower-hope counterparts to the challenge of having children with externalizing disorders, such as ADHD.[28] Horton and Wallander found that, in mothers of children with chronic physical conditions (e.g., cerebral palsy), greater levels of hope were associated with less distress in the face of this significant challenge.[29] Hope is also related to better coping in the context of marital relationships. In one study, more hopeful individuals reported greater marital satisfaction in the face of their partners' advanced breast cancer diagnoses.[30]

Hope's Role in Psychotherapy

Most of us, at some point in our lives, will face difficulties that challenge our ability to pursue our goals. At least in Western society, seeking out counseling or psychotherapy is an important way to address these challenges.

Irving and colleagues found that patients who were higher in hope (i.e., who naturally tend to set these three conditions in their lives) at the beginning of a course of therapy tended to benefit more than their lower-hope counterparts by the end of the therapy.[31]

Although this is good news for people who are already naturally hopeful, what about for those who are not? Fortunately, recent research demonstrates that hope is changeable. Even those with initially low levels of hope can be taught skills for setting the three conditions for hope to thrive.

In one study, for instance, we randomly assigned adults with a variety of mental illness diagnoses to either eight sessions of hope-based group therapy or a waiting list for eight weeks.[32] In this relatively short time, hope-therapy participants showed increases in hope as well as self-esteem and sense of life purpose. Similar results for hope-based therapies have been found in older adults with depression and suicidal ideation, adult survivors of traumatic brain injury, and children in residential care.[33–36]

While these interventions all lasted several weeks or more, much shorter interventions can also affect hope, particularly in people without mental-illness diagnoses. Recently, we tested the efficacy of a single-session, 90-minute hope intervention.[37] College students participated in one of three conditions—a hope workshop, a relaxation-training comparison condition, or a no-treatment control condition. After the study, those in the hope workshop showed greater increases in hope and life purpose than control participants. They also reported greater progress on a self-nominated goal one month later. We furthermore found that those who made the greatest gains in hope during the workshop went on to achieve higher GPAs during the next semester.[38]

Tools for Nurturing Hope

It would be impractical in one chapter to detail all the techniques used in the aforementioned hope-based therapies. However, in the remaining pages, we summarize some of the most important ones, particularly providing guidance for how readers might apply these tools in their own lives. We divide these techniques into three categories—goals, pathways, and agency—with each group of tools designed to help set one of the conditions for hope to thrive.

Tools for Setting Goals

Choosing Goals in Multiple Life Domains

A key to high hope is setting goals in multiple life domains.[7] At any time, it is unlikely that we will be equally successful in all areas of our lives. Just as some investors seek to diversify stock portfolios, it is wise to diversify one's portfolio of goals. By setting goals in different life domains, we can ensure that if a particular set of goals is blocked, there will be other domains of goals to fall back on.[39] Moreover, the increased agency experienced from success in one domain (e.g., fostering new friendships) can help motivate goal pursuit in another, potentially more difficult domain (e.g., finding a romantic partner).

A simple exercise can help to diversify one's goals. Divide a sheet of paper into six boxes any way you would like. At the top of each box, write one of the following: (1) social life, (2) family/home life, (3) romantic life, (4) work life, (5) leisure life, and (6) academic life. (If one of these domains is not personally relevant, just exclude it.) Now, fill in each box with goals you are working on in that domain. These should be medium to large goals (e.g., volunteering for a personally meaningful cause, saving for a vacation, making a new friend); don't write down goals that feel too small to be meaningful. Once you are finished with the list, take a look at your work. There is no need to have goals in every domain, but a diversified mix of at least a few domains is best. Are there any domains that are missing goals? Are you putting too many eggs in one domain's basket? If your goal portfolio seems imbalanced, consider adding goals in one or more domains. You may also consider placing greater emphasis or effort into some of the goals you already have.

Setting Personally Meaningful Goals

As mentioned previously, at least some of our goals should be personally meaningful. Sheldon and colleagues have shown that goals that are consonant with our most important personal values lead to greater well-being than less values-concordant ones.[40,41] Nonetheless, many people spend the bulk of their time pursuing goals that are more important to *others*—their bosses, family members, or friends—than to themselves. Although it's not necessarily unhealthy to do things for other people, it is very easy to forget ourselves in the process.

What do you value most in life? Here are some common values: achievement (success, ambition, intelligence), power (recognition, authority, wealth), pleasure (enjoying life, physical pleasure), stimulation (varied experiences, excitement, adventure), self-direction (independence, creativity, curiosity), social concerns (social justice, environmental justice), relationships (helpfulness, honesty, loyalty), tradition (upholding customs, devotion, humility), dutifulness (self-discipline, politeness, honoring commitments), and security (family security, social order, safety).[42] To further explore your values, take out a sheet of paper, and write your top three values along the left side, with plenty of space between them. Don't feel limited to the ones just mentioned— you can make up your own. Next to each value, write down any goals you are currently working on that allow you to live according to that value. Are at least some of your goals value concordant? If not, consider if you would like to add one or two goals (even small ones) that would allow you to live with greater fidelity to your top values.

Tools for Generating Pathways

Creating Subgoals

Many goals can be large, taking months or even years to accomplish. Such goals can sometimes feel overwhelming unless broken into bite-size pieces. Pathways are often made up of subgoals, or a set of small steps that bring us gradually closer to achieving our big goals.

An important skill involves breaking down goals into this set of much more manageable subgoals. To do this, start by choosing a goal that you would like to break into bite-size pieces. Write that goal at the very top of a sheet of paper. Now, divide the paper into two equal columns. At the top of the first column, write, "What do I need to *have* before I try to achieve this goal?"; at the top of the second column, write, "How do I need to *be* before I try to achieve this goal?" Take a few minutes to record your answers in the appropriate column. Answers to the first question may include commodities like time, money, or training. Answers to the second question may include mental states, like being more outgoing or patient, or physical states, like being healthier or more in shape. Try not to be too hard on yourself while doing this activity. Everyone has skills they could improve or strengths they could focus on gaining. This activity isn't about criticizing yourself but rather about compassionately asking what is needed for you to succeed. Once you have answered these questions, examine what you have written. You have just developed the beginning of a list of subgoals that, if you choose to work on them, could each bring you closer to achieving your goal. In the next activity, you'll arrange them into a plan.

Making a Pathway Map

Some versions of hope therapy have made use of a pathways-mapping exercise to aid participants in planning how to achieve their goals.[32,37,39] For people naturally good at visualizing how they will reach their goals, mapping probably is not necessary. For the rest of us, however, a visual map can help us to more clearly envision the journey ahead.

To make a pathways map, take out a clean sheet of paper and turn it 90 degrees (landscape orientation). Draw a time line across the page. On the left (at the beginning of the time line), write "now"; on the right (at the end of the time line), write a goal you would like to achieve in the next few months to a year. Next, consider the steps that you will need to take (or subgoals) in order to attain this goal; these may include the ones you identified in the previous exercise. Write these along the line in chronological order, jotting down an approximate date of completion next to each one. It is important to note that these dates are not set in stone; they are simply guidelines to aid in planning. It will be best if you do this activity in pencil, so you can erase and rearrange subgoals as needed. One of the important lessons learned from hopeful people is that pathways are never set in stone; it's often necessary and productive to alter them as you encounter obstacles, discover new desires, and learn about yourself along the way.

Tools for Generating Agency

Allowing Yourself to Hope

People are sometimes afraid to hope. When we were children, well-meaning adults may have warned us not to "get our hopes up." We may have been advised not to dream too much, lest we "jinx it." But research has generally failed to show that getting our hopes up exposes us to failure or disappointment.[15] On the contrary, allowing ourselves to get excited about goals is the very essence of agency and provides the motivation necessary to sustain hope and goal-directed activity.[14]

An important way to bolster one's agency involves "hopeful daydreaming."[32,37,39] Similar techniques have been used to increase success in domains including sports, musical performance, and work-skill acquisition, among others.[43–46] Unlike normal fantasy-based daydreaming, in hopeful daydreaming, your task is to close your eyes and envision yourself pursuing each subgoal you wrote on the goal map discussed earlier.[47] Over the course of 10 to 20 minutes, vividly see yourself working on and succeeding at each subgoal, one at a time, then eventually accomplishing your final goal. The key to this exercise is realism, using all five senses. For example, if your goal is to begin cooking more often, you could begin by imagining the first subgoal along your pathway: going shopping for ingredients. Using all five senses, see yourself walking up and down the aisles of your local grocery store, smelling the scents of the various foods, and choosing which ones to purchase. Do the same thing for each subgoal leading to your goal. If you think you might encounter obstacles when working toward any of your subgoals, see yourself encountering and circumnavigating each obstacle with alternative plans.

Talking to Yourself in Hopeful Ways

In large part, agency comes from our beliefs. If we tell ourselves that we are incompetent and cannot accomplish our goals, we are unlikely to try. However, if we tell ourselves that we are competent, we will be more likely to put forth the effort. In other words, the way we talk to ourselves matters. But many of us have a running criticism in our heads that produces such thoughts as "You're stupid," "You're not good enough," "There's no way you'll succeed," or "It's not worth trying." Such self-talk can easily sap our agency.

Though these beliefs may have been internalized at an early age, it's never too late to change them. To begin working on low-agency self-talk, divide a sheet of paper into three columns: "goal," "low-agency self-talk," and "high-agency alternatives." Take a few minutes to write some of the goals in your life in the first column. Once you have done this, consider these goals one by one. What self-talk pops into your mind as you consider each goal? Are you criticizing your chances of achieving this goal? Are you telling yourself you cannot do it? Write this negative self-talk in the second column. Once you've written down your self-talk for a handful of goals, look for patterns. Are there certain phrases that you repeatedly use? These beliefs may be sapping your agency. Last, taking one goal at a time, begin to brainstorm some higher-agency alternatives. For instance, instead of "I can't do this," see if you can tell yourself "I *might* be able to do this, but I won't know unless I try." Be realistic about the difficulties you face. Acknowledging that you face tough obstacles in pursuit of your goal is not low-agency self-talk; it is realistic thinking and can be quite useful. But you can still try to give yourself the message that it is possible to overcome these obstacles.

Revisiting and Revising Your Goals

In addition to "don't get your hopes up," adults often give children a seemingly opposite and equally extreme piece of advice: "*Never* give up." In fact, many people consider a never-give-up attitude synonymous with being a hopeful person. According to research, however, judiciously giving up on certain goals can actually help us to live happy and hopeful lives.[48] Technically referred to as "goal disengagement," it can be healthy to reevaluate your commitment to goals that are either truly blocked or no longer personally meaningful. One reason why goal disengagement may be beneficial is that it frees you to pursue other, previously overlooked goals. If you spend all your energy doggedly pursuing a goal that has outlived its usefulness, you may be missing the opportunity to do other meaningful things. This doesn't mean lowering standards. Quite the contrary: it means valuing your time and energy enough to invest them wisely.

One reason to disengage from a goal is that it's no longer important to you. The natural human tendency is to think we should continue to pursue a goal until it is achieved. Sometimes, however, circumstances can change before we reach that point. When people have difficulty motivating themselves to pursue a goal, sometimes it is because the goal is not as meaningful to them as they originally thought. If you are feeling stagnant in your life, it might be time to reevaluate some of your goals, possibly substituting them for new ones. Take a look at the list of goals you constructed earlier when examining the domains of your life. Is there any goal that does not seem important to you anymore? If yes, ask yourself what the likely outcome of disengaging from that goal would be. If the consequences of disengagement would not be detrimental, consider what new goal or goals you might want to replace it with. The heart of this exercise isn't really disengagement in itself but rather making room in your life for engagement in other more meaningful goals. It is not a good idea to constantly second-guess your goals, of course, so this activity is not one you will want to do often, but a gentle review of your goals every year or two may be just what the doctor ordered.

Conclusion

The Swiss theologian Emil Brunner described hope's role in life as follows: "What oxygen is for the lungs, such is hope for the meaning of human life" (p. 7).[49] But hope doesn't have to be a mysterious or abstract concept. Hope theory offers practical tools to aid in setting the three conditions in our lives under which hope thrives: agency, pathways, and goals.[7,8] Each is dependent on the other, and all three can, in combination, create a positive upward spiral of hopefulness, contributing to our psychological and physical health, personal achievement, and overall well-being.

References

1. Hesiod. (2004). Works and days. In S. M. Trzaskoma, R. S. Smith, & S. Brunet (Eds. & Trans.), *Anthology of classical myth: Primary sources in translation* (pp. 160–167). Indianapolis, IN: Hackett Publishing Company. (Original work published n.d.)

2. Ogden, S. M. (1975). The meaning of Christian hope. *Union Seminary Quarterly Review, 24*, 153–164.

3. Bhikkhu, T. (2006). *Purity of heart: Essays on the Buddhist path.* Valley Center, CA: Metta Forest Monastery.

4. Chödrön, P. (1997). *When things fall apart: Heart advice for difficult times.* Boston, MA: Shambhala Press.

5. Ikeda, D. (2005). Making hope. In K. Krieger & C. Ong (Eds.), *Hold hope, wage peace: Inspiring young leaders to take action for a better world* (pp. 19–22). Santa Barbara, CA: Capra Press.

6. Menninger, K. (1959). The academic lecture on hope. *American Journal of Psychiatry, 109,* 481–491.

7. Snyder, C. R. (1994). *The psychology of hope: You can get there from here.* New York, NY: Free Press.

8. Snyder, C. R. (2002). Hope theory: Rainbows in the mind. *Psychological Inquiry, 13,* 249–275.

9. Piper, W. (1978). *The little engine that could.* New York: Grosset & Dunlap.

10. Alarcon, G. M., Bowling, N. A., & Khazon, S. (2013). Great expectations: A meta-analytic examination of optimism and hope. *Personality and Individual Differences, 54,* 821–827.

11. Feldman, D. B., & Snyder, C. R. (2005). Hope and the meaningful life: Theoretical and empirical associations between goal-directed thinking and life meaning. *Journal of Social and Clinical Psychology, 24,* 401–421.

12. Bailey, T. C., Eng, W., Frisch, M. B., & Snyder, C. R. (2007). Hope and optimism as related to life satisfaction. *Journal of Positive Psychology, 2,* 168–175.

13. Smedema, S. M., Chan, J. Y., & Phillips, B. N. (2014). Core self-evaluations and Snyder's hope theory in persons with spinal cord injuries. *Rehabilitation Psychology, 59,* 399–406.

14. Feldman, D. B., Rand, K. L., & Kahle-Wrobleski, K. (2009). Hope and goal attainment: Testing a basic prediction of hope therapy. *Journal of Social and Clinical Psychology, 28,* 479–497.

15. Snyder, C. R., Rand, K. L., King, E. A., Feldman, D. B., & Woodward, J. T. (2002). "False" hope. *Journal of Clinical Psychology, 58,* 1003–1022.

16. Lewis, H. A., & Kliewer, W. (1996). Hope, coping, and adjustment among children with sickle cell disease: Tests of mediator and moderator models. *Journal of Pediatric Psychology, 21,* 25–41.

17. Chang, E. C., Martos, T., Sallay, V., Chang, O. D., Wright, K. M., Najarian, A. S. M., & Lee, J. (2017). Examining optimism and hope as protective factors of suicide risk in Hungarian college students: Is risk highest among those lacking positive psychological protection? *Cognitive Therapy and Research, 41,* 278–288.

18. Marques, S. C., Pais-Riberio, J. L., & Lopez, S. J. (2011). The role of positive psychology constructs in predicting mental health and academic achievement in Portuguese children and adolescents: A two-year longitudinal study. *Journal of Happiness Studies, 12,* 1049–1062.

19. Rand, K. L., Martin, A. D., & Shea, A. M. (2011). Hope, but not optimism predicts academic performance of law students beyond previous academic achievement. *Journal of Research in Personality, 45,* 683–686.

20. Snyder, C. R., Shorey, H. S., Cheavens, J., Pulvers, K. M., Adams, V. H., & Wiklund, C. (2002). Hope and academic success in college. *Journal of Educational Psychology, 94,* 820–826.

21. Gallagher, M. W., Marques, S. C., & Lopez, S. J. (2017). Hope and the academic trajectory of college students. *Journal of Happiness Studies, 18,* 341–352.

22. Buckelew, S. P., Crittendon, R. S., Butkovic, J. D., Price, K. B., & Hurst, M. (2008). Hope as a predictor of academic performance. *Psychological Reports, 103,* 411–414.

23. Curry, L., Snyder, C. R., Cook, D. L., Ruby, B. C., & Rehm, M. (1997). Role of hope in academic and sports achievement. *Journal of Personality and Social Psychology, 73,* 1257–1267.

24. Feldman, D. B., & Kubota, M. (2015). Hope, self-efficacy, optimism, and academic achievement: Constructs and levels of specificity in predicting college grade-point average. *Learning and Individual Differences, 37,* 210–216.

25. Marques, S. C., Lopez, S. J., Fontaine, A. M., Coimbra, S., & Mitchell, J. (2015). How much hope is enough? Levels of hope and students' psychological and school functioning. *Psychology in the Schools, 52,* 325–334.

26. Valle, M. F., Huebner, E. S., & Suldo, S. M. (2006). An analysis of hope as a psychological strength. *Journal of School Psychology, 44,* 393–406.

27. Hirschi, A. (2014). Hope as a resource for self-directed career management: Investigating mediating effects on proactive career behaviors and life and job satisfaction. *Journal of Happiness Studies, 15,* 1495–1512.

28. Kashdan, T. B., Pelham, W. E., Lang, A. R., Hoza, B., Jacob, R. G., Jennings, J. R., . . . Gnagy, E. M. (2002). Hope and optimism as human strengths in parents of children with externalizing disorders: Stress is in the eye of the beholder. *Journal of Social and Clinical Psychology, 21,* 441–468.

29. Horton, T. V., & Wallander, J. L. (2001). Hope and social support as resilience factors against psychological distress of mothers who care for children with chronic physical conditions. *Rehabilitation Psychology, 46,* 382–399.

30. Rock, E. E., Steiner, J. L., Rand, K. L., & Bigatti, S. M. (2014). Dyadic influence of hope and optimism on patient marital satisfaction among couples with advanced breast cancer. *Supportive Care in Cancer, 22,* 2351–2359.

31. Irving, L. M., Snyder, C. R., Cheavens, J., Gravel, L., Hanke, J., Hilberg, P., & Nelson, N. (2004). The relationship between hope and outcomes at the pretreatment, beginning, and later phases of psychotherapy. *Journal of Psychotherapy Integration, 14,* 419–443.

32. Cheavens, J. S., Feldman, D. B., Gum, A., Michael, S. T., & Snyder, C. R. (2006). Hope theory in a community sample: A pilot investigation. *Social Indicators Research, 77,* 61–78.

33. Klausner, E. J., Clarkin, J. F., Spielman, L., Pudo, C., Abrams, R., & Alexopoulos, G. S. (1998). Late-life depression and functional disability: The role of goal-focused group psychotherapy. *International Journal of Geriatric Psychiatry, 13,* 707–716.

34. Lapierre, S., Dubé, M., Bouffard, L., & Alain, M. (2007). Addressing suicidal ideations through the realization of meaningful personal goals. *Crisis, 28,* 16–25.

35. Wilbur, R. C., & Parenté, R. (2008). A cognitive technology for fostering hope. *Cognitive Technology, 13,* 24–29.

36. McNeal, R., Handwerk, M. L., Field, C. E., Roberts, M. C., Soper, S., Huefner, J. C., . . . Ringle, J. L. (2006). Hope as an outcome variable among youths in a residential care setting. *American Journal of Orthopsychiatry, 76,* 304–311.

37. Feldman, D. B., & Dreher, D. E. (2012). Can hope be changed in 90 minutes? Testing the efficacy of a single-session goal-pursuit intervention for college students. *Journal of Happiness Studies, 13,* 745–759.

38. Davidson, O. B., Feldman, D. B., & Margalit, M. (2012). A focused intervention for 1st-year college students: Promoting hope, sense of coherence, and self-efficacy. *The Journal of Psychology, 14,* 333–352.

39. McDermott, D., & Snyder, C. R. (1999). *Making hope happen.* Oakland, CA: New Harbinger.

40. Sheldon, K. M. (2001). The self-concordance model of healthy goal-striving: Implications for well-being and personality development. In P. Schmuck & K. M. Sheldon (Eds.), *Life goals and well-being: Towards a positive psychology of human striving* (pp. 17–35). Seattle, WA: Hogrefe & Huber Publishers.

41. Sheldon, K. M., & Elliot, A. J. (1999). Goal striving, need satisfaction, and longitudinal well-being: The self-concordance model. *Journal of Personality and Social Psychology, 76,* 482–497.

42. Schwartz, S. H. (1992). Universals in the content and structure of values: Theoretical advances and empirical tests in 20 countries. *Advances in Experimental Social Psychology, 25,* 1–65.

43. Feltz, D. L., & Landers, D. M. (1983). The effects of mental practice on motor skill learning and performance: A meta-analysis. *Journal of Sport Psychology, 5,* 25–57.

44. Murphy, S. M. (1990). Models of imaginary in sport psychology: A review. *Journal of Mental Imagery, 14,* 153–172.

45. Lim, S., & Lippman, L. G. (1991). Mental practice and memorization of piano music. *The Journal of General Psychology, 118,* 21–30.

46. Wohldmann, E. L., Healy, A. F., & Bourne, L. E., Jr. (2008). A mental practice superiority effect: Less retroactive interference and more transfer than physical practice. *Journal of Experimental Psychology: Learning, Memory, and Cognition, 34,* 823–833.

47. Oettingen, G., & Mayer, D. (2002). The motivating function of thinking about the future: Expectations versus fantasies. *Journal of Personality and Social Psychology, 83,* 1198–1212.

48. Wrosch, C., Scheier, M. F., Miller, G. E., Schulz, R., & Carver, C. S. (2003). Adaptive self-regulation of unattainable goals: Goal disengagement, goal reengagement, and subjective well-being. *Personality and Social Psychology Bulletin, 29,* 1494–1508.

49. Beasley-Murray, G. R. (2006). *The coming of God: The Emanuel Ajahi Dahunsi memorial New Testament lectures 1981.* Eugene, OR: Wipf and Stock Publishers.

CHAPTER THREE

Mindfulness and Health: Evidence-Based and Clinical Applications

Shauna L. Shapiro and Sophie von Garnier

As we attempt to scale mindfulness and integrate it into Western science, culture, and society, it is necessary to bring great sensitivity and care to its definition. While it is crucial to illustrate mindfulness in ways that are universally applicable, and which transcend religion and culture, we must also find ways to stay rooted in its deep transformational essence. Often, in our attempts to create a simple, digestible definition of mindfulness, we reduce it to a unidimensional construct, for example, a cognitive attentional process, and potentially miss its rich and multifaceted nature.[1]

Thus, the first intention of this chapter is to explore the question, "What is mindfulness?" In doing so, we offer a multidimensional model of mindfulness that is universally applicable and yet still retains the deep wisdom and heart of the practice. We will then explore a secondary question, "Is mindfulness helpful?" and review the clinical applications of mindfulness, focusing on three subject areas: (1) physiological medical conditions, (2) psychological diagnostic disorders, and (3) prevention and healthy stressed populations.

What Is Mindfulness?

Given that mindfulness is nonconceptual, nonlinear, and deeply paradoxical in nature, attempting to create a linear conceptual definition is problematic. And yet, if we are to integrate mindfulness into mainstream culture, science, medicine, education, psychology, and so on, we need to have a coherent, mutually agreed upon definition.

Although the concept of mindfulness is most often associated with Buddhism, its phenomenological nature is embedded in most religious and spiritual traditions as well as Western philosophical and psychological schools of thought.[2,3] And yet, mindfulness is a universal human capacity that transcends culture and religion. Mindfulness is an inherent aspect of being human, a state of awareness accessible to us all. Thus, we define mindfulness as "the awareness that arises through intentionally attending in an open, caring, and discerning way."[4]

This awareness involves a *knowing* and *experiencing* of life as it arises and passes away each moment. It is a way of relating to all experience—positive, negative, and neutral—in an open, kind, and receptive way. This awareness involves freedom from grasping and wanting anything to be different. It simply knows what is truly here because it allows us to see the nature of reality clearly and with compassion, without all our conditioned patterns of perceiving clouding our awareness.

Mindfulness does not necessarily change our experience; it simply adds the resonance of awareness to experience so we can know it deeply and intimately. Ultimately, mindful awareness is about seeing things as they are so that we can respond consciously and skillfully.

Although mindful awareness is inherent in everyone, it is often hidden by deep conditioning—our parents, teachers, relationships, and society have influenced us in ways known and unknown. Our patterns have become so ingrained that we may not realize we are engaging in them. We often live on autopilot, being pushed and pulled by our patterns, not fully awake and free to the reality of the present moment. To counteract this conditioning, we can train our mind in the ability to be with and *know* our experience as it arises and passes. This requires sustained practice, the intentional training of our mind to pay attention in a kind, discerning way. We call this training mindfulness practice.

In an attempt to elucidate both the simplicity and complexity of mindful practice, we developed a model of mindfulness comprised of three core elements: intention, attention, and attitude.[5] Intention, attention, and attitude are not separate processes or stages—they are interwoven aspects of a single cyclic *process* and occur simultaneously, the three elements informing and feeding back into each other. Mindful practice *is* this moment-to-moment process.

Intention is simply knowing why we are practicing mindfulness meditation, what our aspirations and motivations are for practice. As Kabat-Zinn writes, "Your intentions set the stage for what is possible. They remind you from moment to moment of why you are practicing in the first place" (p. 32).[6] He continues, "I used to think that meditation practice was so powerful . . . that as long as you did it at all, you would see growth and change. But time has taught me that some kind of personal vision is also necessary" (p. 46).[6] Intentions are not outcome-based goals one actively strives toward during each meditation practice. Instead, they are a direction, setting the compass of our heart in the direction we want to head.

A second fundamental component of mindfulness is *attention*. In the context of mindful practice, paying attention involves observing the operations of one's moment-to-moment internal and external experience. This is what Husserl (p. 168) refers to as going "back to the 'things themselves,'" that is, suspending (and/or noting) all the ways of interpreting experience and attending to experience itself as it presents itself in the here and now.[7] In this way, one learns to attend not only to the surrounding world but also to the *contents* of one's consciousness, moment by moment.

Mindful practice involves a dynamic process of learning how to cultivate attention that is discerning and nonreactive, sustained and concentrated, so that we can see clearly what is arising in the present moment (including our emotional reactions, if that is what arises). As Germer notes, "An unstable mind is like an unstable camera; we get a fuzzy picture" (p. 16).[8]

The *attitude* with which we pay attention is also essential. According to Kabat-Zinn, mindfulness is understood "not just as a bare attention but as an *affectionate* [italics added] attention" (p. 5).[9] This attitudinal dimension of mindfulness, which involves a kind, open, discerning attitude, must be explicitly introduced as part of the practice. Attending without bringing the attitudinal qualities into the practice may result in practice that is condemning or judgmental of inner (or outer) experience. Such an approach may well have consequences contrary to the intentions of the practice, for example, cultivating patterns of judgment and striving instead of equanimity and acceptance. The field of neuroplasticity demonstrates that our repeated experiences shape our brain. If we continually practice meditation with a cold, judgmental, and impatient attention, these are the pathways that will get stronger. Our intention instead is to practice with an attitude of open, caring attention.

The attitudinal qualities do not add anything to the experience itself but rather infuse the holding space of attention with acceptance, openness, caring, and curiosity. For example, if, while practicing mindfulness, impatience arises, the impatience is noted with acceptance and kindness. However, these qualities are not meant to be substituted for the impatience or to make the impatience disappear; they are simply the container. The attitudes are not an attempt to make things be a certain way; they are an attempt to relate to whatever is in a certain way.[6]

With intentional training, one becomes increasingly able to cultivate attitudes of patience, compassion, and openness and infuse them into the attentional practice. Present moment attention occurs within a context of gentleness, kindness, and acceptance.

A Context of Interdependence

Implicit in this model is the worldview of interdependence, which has always been an inherent dimension of mindfulness and provides an essential context for the practice. We define interdependence as the understanding that nothing is separate, that we live in a complexly interwoven system where everything affects everything else. Interdependence is not just some lofty spiritual ideal; it is a founding principle of ecology, cybernetics, physics, culture, and systems theory.[10,11]

This concept of interdependence is at the heart of the traditional Buddhist teachings, from which mindfulness arose. This worldview in traditional Buddhist texts is referred to as interdependent coarising—the understanding that all things arise based on causes and conditions and that nothing happens in isolation.[12] Everything is connected. This view of interdependence is not solely Buddhist and is seen across various perennial wisdom traditions, religions, and philosophies.

Mindfulness, therefore, can be defined as intentionally paying attention with an attitude of kindness and discernment and within a context of interdependence. Mindfulness is an inherent human capacity, and it is a practice that can be cultivated and strengthened. Fundamentally, mindfulness is a way of being.

Is Mindfulness Helpful?

Now that we have explored the question "What is mindfulness?" we turn our attention to the next question, "Is mindfulness helpful?" In the following, we present a summary of the most salient and rigorous mindfulness research across three main categories: (1) physiological medical conditions, (2) psychological diagnostic disorders, and (3) prevention and healthy stressed populations.

Physiological Medical Conditions

Four decades of research have demonstrated the beneficial effects of mindfulness-based interventions across a wide range of disorders. For example, mindfulness-based stress-reduction intervention (MBSR) and mindfulness-based cognitive therapy (MBCT), which combines elements of cognitive-behavioral therapy (CBT) with MBSR, have been shown to help manage pain, anxiety, and depressive symptoms associated with physical conditions, including diabetes, epilepsy, fibromyalgia, and vascular disease.[13–19] Below we highlight some of the most current research.

Pain Management

A recent meta-analysis by Goyal and colleagues investigating randomized controlled studies (RCTs) with active controls found moderate evidence (Cohen's $d = 0.33$) that mindfulness interventions can help alleviate pain.[20] Veehof and colleagues reviewed 25 RCTs that used either MBSR, MBCT, or acceptance and commitment therapy—a therapeutic intervention that integrates mindfulness and acceptance with goal commitment and behavior change—in their efficacy in treating chronic pain.[4,15,21] Examining the impact of these interventions, the researchers found small, yet significant, effects for increases in quality of life; decreases in pain intensity, disability, and depression; and moderate effects for pain interference and anxiety at postintervention. These encouraging results regarding pain interference suggest that while actual pain reduction might be small, patients successfully apply the mindfulness techniques they have learned, increasing their capacity to better live with and manage chronic pain.

Cancer

Besides chronic pain, one illness that has garnered much attention from mindfulness researchers is cancer. Ledesma and Kumano conducted a meta-analysis with both observational and randomized studies and found a medium effect size ($d = 0.48$) for the mental benefits of mindfulness-based interventions (MBI) for cancer patients and a small effect size ($d = 0.18$) for the effects of MBI on physical health.[22] Researchers have found that physiological benefits of mindfulness-based treatment programs include decreases in the stress hormone cortisol, maintaining telomere length, and faster recovery of immune cell functioning.[23–25]

We will now review research examining psychological outcomes of MBI for cancer treatment. Piet, Würtzen, and Zachariae found in a meta-analysis of nine RTC studies employing mindfulness therapies for cancer patients and survivors that treatment recipients showed clinically significant decreases in both anxiety ($d = 0.37$) and depressive symptoms ($d = 0.44$).[26] Carlson and colleagues also found that those distressed breast-cancer patients who were randomly assigned to a mindfulness-based cancer recovery group saw a greater reduction of stress symptoms than women in supportive expressive group therapy or a minimal-intervention control group and a greater increase in quality of life than women in the control group.[27,28]

Promising results are also coming from the area of remote mindfulness therapy via the Internet, which can enable patients to access treatment even if they live in rural areas or find it difficult to leave their home. Bruggeman-Everts and colleagues designed a nine-week, three-armed RTC comparing what is known as ambulant activity feedback (AAF) with an e-version of MBCT for an unguided active control group.[29] In comparison to the active control group, participants in both the AAF and the eMBCT conditions reported significant decreases in the severity of their chronic cancer-related fatigue.

While these studies and meta-analyses support the idea that mindfulness techniques can be used as a valuable intervention for cancer patients, mental-health professionals and physicians should be aware that mindfulness interventions might not be appropriate for all such patients. A recent randomized-controlled study compared a physically focused relaxation therapy approach with a brief mindfulness-based intervention to reduce distress in patients undergoing chemotherapy.[30] The results showed that, in this specific context of acute cancer treatment, the physical-relaxation techniques might be preferable, as participants in the mindfulness condition reported an increase in symptom distress and a marginal increase in social avoidance as well as a decrease in reported quality of life. The participants in the physical-relaxation condition either stayed the same or improved on these measures. While numerous studies have examined mindfulness's effects on medical conditions and related psychopathologies, we need further research, especially employing RCTs, to identify in which circumstances mindfulness approaches are most efficacious.

Psychological Diagnostic Disorders

Research suggests that mindfulness interventions can not only help alleviate anxiety and depressive symptoms that accompany physiological medical conditions but can also play a role in decreasing the symptomology of a wide variety of psychological disorders, including depression, anxiety, borderline personality disorder, binge-eating disorder, substance-use disorder, and posttraumatic stress disorder.[31–35] While there are promising findings for the treatment of many of these disorders using mindfulness practices, the most effectively treated across a wide variety of meta-analyses are anxiety and depression.[20,36] Research has also demonstrated that mindfulness practices presented as a subcomponent of a therapy model, rather than its core element, can strongly contribute to treatment success, as seen in the treatment of borderline personality disorder.[37]

Depression

MBCT, which was originally developed to prevent depression relapse, has also been shown to be effective for patients who are currently depressed.[38,39] When Goyal and colleagues investigated the effect sizes for reducing depressive symptoms using mindfulness interventions in RCTs with active controls, they found a small to moderate clinically significant effect size ($d = 0.30$) after eight weeks and a small but clinically significant effect size ($d = 0.22$) three to six months following the intervention.[20] Similarly, Williams and colleagues found in a three-armed RCT that while MBCT was on par with treatment as usual and CBT for patients with recurrent depression, MBCT was more effective for those who had experienced childhood trauma.[39] Kuyken and colleagues came to a similar conclusion.[40] While MBCT did not outperform maintenance pharmacotherapy using antidepressants, depressed patients with a history of childhood abuse showed lower relapse rates. MBCT has also proven helpful to patients who are in an active episode or suffer from chronic depression.[41] Eisendrath and colleagues explored whether an eight-week MBCT intervention in combination with pharmacotherapy might be able to interrupt lengthy episodes of treatment-resistant depression in comparison to a randomized active control group also receiving pharmacotherapy but participating in a health-enhancement program (including physical fitness and music therapy) instead.[31] As hypothesized, participants in the MBCT group experienced a significantly greater reduction in the severity of their symptoms.

Anxiety

As with depression, mindfulness has been shown to help reduce anxiety, not only when co-occurring with medical conditions but also without comorbidities. In their comprehensive meta-analysis, Goyal and colleagues found small to moderate clinically significant effect sizes for mindfulness interventions on anxiety ranging from 0.38 after eight weeks (after the intervention has been completed) to 0.22 after three to six months.[20] While Kabat-Zinn and colleagues were the first to successfully treat anxiety disorders with MBSR, later studies have implemented more rigorous experimental designs, using RTCs and active control groups to investigate if MBSR's effects are strong enough to compete with more established therapies, such as CBT.[42] Researchers including Koszycki, Benger, Shlik, and Brandwein, as well as Goldin and colleagues, compared MBSR to cognitive-behavioral group therapy (CBGT) for generalized social anxiety disorder (SAD).[32,43] Goldin and colleagues also included a waitlist control condition in their RCT design. Each research group came to the conclusion that MBSR and CBGT are both effective in improving functionality of patients. Koszycki and colleagues' study revealed that patients leaving either program had greater functionality, better mood, and greater quality of life compared to baseline. In Goldin and colleagues' study, both were equally successful at reducing social anxiety symptoms (except for CBGT's better capacity to reduce subtle avoidance behaviors), a finding that was contrary to Koszycki and colleagues' earlier study that found CBGT to be superior in terms of reducing SAD severity.[32,43]

Borderline Personality Disorder

While working with patients struggling with anxiety and depression can be very challenging for clinicians, treating personality disorders successfully is famously difficult because such disorders are often not only deeply ingrained into a patient's identity but also have often gone untreated for years. One of the most prominent and challenging personality disorders to live with (both for the patients and their loved ones) is borderline personality disorder (BPD). Symptoms of BPD include fear of abandonment, impulsivity, interpersonal conflict, increased difficulty in dealing with intense negative emotions, and an unstable identity.[44] One of the most widely practiced evidence-based treatments for BPD is dialectical behavior therapy (DBT).[45,46] DBT is a multifaceted approach that includes individual counseling, telephone coaching by the patient's therapist, group skills training, and mindfulness training. When comparing 30 patients who had been diagnosed with BPD to 30 control participants from the general population, Marzal and Górska found that the higher patients scored on BPD symptomology, the lower they scored on mindfulness.[47] As was expected, an increase in BPD was highly correlated with an increase in emotion dysregulation. When Panos and colleagues investigated the effectiveness of DBT in treating borderline personality disorder in five RCTs, they found that while DBT was not significantly better at treating depressive symptoms compared to treatment as usual, it was marginally better at reducing attrition from the treatment program and significantly better at decreasing parasuicidal and suicidal behaviors.[48] The latter is a crucial finding given that BPD is often comorbid with self-harming behaviors.[44] Pano and colleagues' study results correspond well with Öst's review and meta-analysis of 13 RCTs, of which 9 were studies using DBT, almost exclusively for BPD patients.[37,48] Öst found a significant medium effect size ($d = 0.58$) for DBT treatments, which is an encouraging finding for both patients and mental health professionals alike.

More recently, Meyers and colleagues have investigated if veterans who show comorbidities of BPD and PTSD could be successfully treated using DBT together with the gold-standard treatment for PTSD, prolonged-exposure therapy (PE).[33] The results of their pilot study suggest they might: while the decreases in dysfunctional coping styles and PTSD were rather small, Meyers and colleagues found a moderate decrease in suicide ideation ($d = 0.64$). Given that in 2016 alone, we lost 20 veterans each day to suicide, we have no time to lose to develop and validate the most effective treatment options possible.[49]

Prevention and Healthy Stressed Populations

Mindfulness training can also be utilized to mitigate risks for developing psychopathologies in healthy individuals.

Mindfulness Interventions as Prevention Tools

Given that early signs of psychological distress can be predictors for later mental-health issues in adulthood—and that some promising findings suggest that mindfulness might be a protective factor against the negative effects of stress—parents, educators, and mental-health professionals are eager to reach children and adolescents as early as possible.[50] However, rigidly conducted experimental interventions are still sparse.[51] Britton and colleagues designed and investigated the impacts of a teacher-taught, six-week daily mindfulness-based classroom intervention on well-being in sixth graders and compared results with an active control group.[52] Interestingly, both groups saw an equal increase in positive affect and declines in clinical symptoms, such as difficulties with attention, internalizing and externalizing problems, and negative affect. Neither treatment group saw an increase in self-reported mindfulness. However, the mindfulness group saw a greater decrease in the development of thoughts and behaviors related to self-harm and suicidality than the students in the active control group. Another RCT waitlist-control intervention designed for fourth and fifth graders in an urban public school revealed positive effects of a 12-week mindfulness and yoga intervention, including a decrease in rumination, emotional arousal, and intrusive thoughts among students in the treatment group.[53] In addition, a recent meta-analysis examined 20 mindfulness interventions for children and adolescents, 16 with nonclinical youth and 4 with youth with diagnosed psychological disorders.[54] The overall effect size for mindfulness interventions was small ($d = 0.24$) yet significant and showed an advantage over active control conditions.

Mindfulness interventions remain helpful when moving into adulthood. In a recent narrative review study analyzing 57 studies of mindfulness interventions in college, three main findings stood out: students experienced a decrease in self-reported stress and anxiety and an increase in mindfulness.[55] Furthermore, a meta-analysis that examined 29 controlled and uncontrolled studies on the effects of MBSR with healthy adults found a small effect of mindfulness interventions on burnout; moderate effects on decreasing anxiety, depression, and stress; and moderate effects on increasing quality of life.[56] While these studies are encouraging, more research is needed in order to understand the extent to which mindfulness can prevent psychological disorders across the life span.

Mindful Romantic Relationships

While few things can bring the joy and vitality a loving romantic relationship can provide, unfortunately, if relationships turn sour, they can become great stressors in both partners' lives. Being more mindful might not only make someone a better partner, but bringing mindfulness techniques into the couple's life may be beneficial as well.[57, 58] Several studies have shown that trait mindfulness is associated with numerous behaviors that contribute to more satisfying relationships, including a better ability to not only recognize but also to communicate emotions, more adaptive response skills when facing relationship conflict, and being more empathetic toward one's partner.[57, 59] The findings of a recent study with 127 heterosexual couples suggest that one of the factors that might contribute to higher relationship satisfaction among couples with higher trait mindfulness is perceived partner responsiveness.[60] Adair and colleagues found that partners who scored higher in trait mindfulness' "acting with awareness" subscale were perceived by their significant other as more responsive to their concerns, which subsequently correlated with higher relationship satisfaction.[60, 61]

Given these promising findings, it is not surprising that mindfulness techniques have been implemented in various approaches to couples therapy. One such approach, mindfulness-based relationship enhancement, has been tested with 44 generally satisfied heterosexual couples in a RCT with a waitlist control group.[58] This eight-week course adapted many mindfulness techniques to couples therapy, including partner yoga, a dyadic eye-gazing exercise, a mindful touch and movement exercise, mindful communication behaviors, and practicing loving-kindness meditation while sending loving thoughts to one's partner. The researchers found an increase in relationship satisfaction and coping skills and a decrease in relationship distress. A follow-up analysis found that these effects were mediated by the couple's sense of self-expansion during these shared mindfulness exercises.[62] Another therapeutic approach that has formally integrated mindfulness techniques into couples' work is pragmatic-experimental therapy for couples, which includes exercises to help the couple relate to distressing emotions during conflict more mindfully, use breathing and sensory exercises to interrupt rumination, and practice mindful self-soothing.[63] While these approaches show promise, further research, specifically utilizing randomized-control trials, is needed to gain more knowledge into how these and other approaches work with couples in distress.

Conclusions and Directions for Future Research

The past four decades have seen an exponential increase in mindfulness research across a wide range of populations and settings. The results have been quite promising, and yet there are multiple directions for future research. One of the most important areas for future study and attention is the inclusion of diverse and underrepresented populations, including those of various socioeconomic statuses, education levels, ethnicities, races, and gender identifications. We need to explore with great sensitivity and rigor as to how to bring these concepts out of the ivory tower and investigate if and how they can benefit individuals who are not part of the less-diverse samples typically studied in the social sciences.

We also strive for future research to utilize the most rigorous methodologies, including multitrait, multimethod assessments, to explore the subtle yet significant changes that can occur through mindfulness practice. In particular, it will be important to combine objective physiological data, first-person narrative introspective data, and third-party observational ratings. The combined perspectives will complement our findings and offer a more unified and integrative understanding. We also need measures to assess health from a systems perspective, an assessment sensitive to the multiple levels of health.

Finally, we suggest studying the impact of teaching mindfulness within a context of interdependence. Western science and academia have steered away from this idea in our attempt to make mindfulness more easily digestible in the West. This "decontextualizing" of mindfulness from its religious and cultural roots has been essential to its integration in the West. And yet, nothing can ever be truly decontextualized. In actuality, we have "recontextualized" mindfulness within a reductionist, dualistic context. This Western conception of mindfulness often characterizes it simply as a tool for "stress management," focusing on symptom alleviation instead of acknowledging the larger process from a systems perspective, which may prevent the individual from achieving "optimal health," defined by the World Health Organization (1946) as more than the absence of disease and involving mental, physical, and social well-being.[64, 65] Such a reductionist model cannot address all the multilevel phenomena that create and sustain optimal health. The goal is not simply to return physiological indicators of health to normal levels. While there is nothing wrong with using meditation to lower blood pressure, for example, we suggest that mindfulness practice explicitly taught from the theoretical perspective of interdependence may be more effective at promoting healing on a systemic level as well as on a symptom level.

If we are to bring a connected and integrative approach to health, we need to approach health systemically and comprehensively. As Kabat-Zinn writes, "Science is searching for more comprehensive models that are truer to our understanding of the interconnectedness of space and time, mass and energy, mind and body, even consciousness and the universe" (p. 151).[6]

References

1. Brown, K. W., & Ryan, R. M. (2003). The benefits of being present: Mindfulness and its   role in psychological well-being. *Journal of Personality and Social Psychology, 84,* 822–848.

2. Brown, K. W., & Cordon, S. (2009). Toward a phenomenology of mindfulness: Subjective experience and emotional correlates. In F. Didonna (Ed.), *Clinical handbook of mindfulness* (pp. 59–91). New York: Springer-Verlag.

3. Walsh, R. (2000). *Essential spirituality: The 7 central practices to awaken heart and mind.* New York: Wiley.

4. Shapiro, S. L., & Carlson, L. E. (2017). *The art and science of mindfulness: Integrating mindfulness into psychology and the helping professions* (2nd ed.). Washington, DC: American Psychological Association.

5. Shapiro, S. L., Carlson, L. E., Astin, J. A., & Freedman, B. (2006). Mechanisms of mindfulness. *Journal of Clinical Psychology, 62,* 373–386.

6. Kabat-Zinn, J. (1990). *Full catastrophe living: Using the wisdom of your body and mind to face stress, pain, and illness.* New York: Delacorte Press.

7. Husserl, E. (2001). *Logical investigations* (Vols. 1 and 2) (J. N. Findlay, Trans.) (D. Moran, Ed.). New York: Routledge. (Original work published 1900 & 1901)

8. Germer, C. K. (2005). Mindfulness: What is it? What does it matter? In C. K. Germer, R. D. Siegel, & P. R. Fulton (Eds.), *Mindfulness and psychotherapy* (pp. 3–27). New York: The Guilford Press.

9. Cullen, M. (2006). Mindfulness: The heart of the Buddhist meditation? A conversation with Joseph Goldstein, Jon Kabat-Zinn, and Alan Wallace. *Inquiring Mind: A Semiannual Journal of the Vipassana Community, 22,* 4–7.

10. Mulej, M. (2007). Systems theory: A worldview and/or a methodology aimed at requisite holism/realism of humans' thinking, decisions, and action. *Systems Research and Behavioral Science, 24,* 347–357.

11. Nakano, S., & Murakami, M. (2001). Reciprocal subsidies: Dynamic interdependence between terrestrial and aquatic food webs. *Proceedings of the National Academy of Sciences, 98,* 166–170.

12. Nhat Hanh, T. (1998). *The heart of the Buddha's teaching: Transforming suffering into peace, joy, and liberation.* New York: Harmony Books.

13. Kabat-Zinn, J., Lipworth, L., & Burney, R. (1985). The clinical use of mindfulness meditation for the self-regulation of chronic pain. *Journal of Behavioral Medicine, 8,* 163–190.

14. Segal, Z. V., Williams, M. G., & Teasdale, J. D. (2002). *Mindfulness-based cognitive therapy for depression: A new approach to preventing relapse.* New York: Guilford Press.

15. Veehof, M. M., Trompetter, H. R., Bohlmeijer, E. T., & Schreurs, K. M. G. (2016). Acceptance- and mindfulness-based interventions for the treatment of chronic pain: A meta-analytic review. *Cognitive Behaviour Therapy, 45,* 5–31.

16. Van Son, J., Nyklíček, I., Pop, V. J., Blonk, M. C., Erdtsieck, R. J., & Pouwer, F. (2014). Mindfulness-based cognitive therapy for people with diabetes and emotional problems: Long-term follow-up findings from the DiaMind randomized controlled trial. *Journal of Psychosomatic Research, 77,* 81–84.

17. Thompson, N. J., Patel, A. H., Selwa, L. M., Stoll, S. C., Begley, C. E., Johnson, E. K., & Fraser, R. T. (2015). Expanding the efficacy of project UPLIFT: Distance delivery of mindfulness-based depression prevention to people with epilepsy. *Journal of Consulting and Clinical Psychology, 83,* 304–313.

18. Lauche, R., Cramer, H., Dobos, G., Langhorst, J., & Schmidt, S. (2013). A systematic review and meta-analysis of mindfulness-based stress reduction for the fibromyalgia syndrome. *Journal of Psychosomatic Research, 75,* 500–510.

19. Abbott, R. A., Whear, R., Rodgers, L. R., Bethel, A., Coon, J. T., Kuyken, W., . . . Dickens, C. (2014). Effectiveness of mindfulness-based stress reduction and mindfulness-based cognitive therapy in vascular disease: A systematic review and meta-analysis of randomised controlled trials. *Journal of Psychosomatic Research, 76,* 341–351.

20. Goyal, M., Singh, S., Sibinga, E. M. S., Gould, N. F., Rowland-Seymour, A., Sharma, R., . . . Haythornthwaite, J. A. (2014). Meditation programs for psychological stress and well-being: A systematic review and meta-analysis. *JAMA Internal Medicine, 174,* 357–368.

21. Hayes, S. C., Luoma, J. B., Bond, F. W., Masuda, A., & Lillis, J. (2006). Acceptance and commitment therapy: Model, processes and outcomes. *Behaviour Research and Therapy, 44,* 1–25.

22. Ledesma, D., & Kumano, H. (2009). Mindfulness-based stress reduction and cancer: A meta-analysis. *Psycho-Oncology, 18,* 571–579.

23. Carlson, L. E., Speca, M., Faris, P., & Patel, K. D. (2007). One year prepost intervention follow-up of psychological, immune, endocrine and blood pressure outcomes of mindfulness-based stress reduction (MBSR) in breast and prostate cancer outpatients. *Brain, Behavior, and Immunity, 21,* 1038–1049.

24. Carlson, L. E., Beattie, T. L., Giese-Davis, J., Faris, P., Tamagawa, R., Fick, L. J., . . . Speca, M. (2015). Mindfulness-based cancer recovery and supportive expressive therapy (SET) maintain telomere length relative to control in distressed breast cancer survivors. *Cancer, 121,* 476–484.

25. Lengacher, C. A., Kip, K. E., Barta, M., Post-White, J., Fitzgerald, S., Newton, C., Barta, M., . . . Klein, T. W. (2013). Lymphocyte recovery after breast cancer treatment and mindfulness-based stress reduction (MBSR) therapy. *Biological Research for Nursing, 15,* 37–47.

26. Piet, J., Würtzen, H., & Zachariae, R. (2012). The effect of mindfulness-based therapy on symptoms of anxiety and depression in adult cancer patients and survivors: A systematic review and meta-analysis. *Journal of Consulting and Clinical Psychology, 80,* 1007–1020.

27. Carlson, L. E., Doll, R., Stephen, J., Faris, P., Tamagawa, R., Drysdale, E., & Speca, M. (2013). Randomized controlled trial of mindfulness-based cancer recovery versus supportive expressive group therapy for distressed survivors of breast cancer (MINDSET). *Journal of Clinical Oncology, 31,* 3119–3126.

28. Carlson, L. E., & Speca, M. (2010). *Mindfulness-based cancer recovery: A step-by-step MBSR approach to help you cope with treatment and reclaim your life.* Oakland, CA: New Harbinger.

29. Bruggeman-Everts, F. Z., Wolvers, M. D. J., van de Schoot, R., Vollenbroek-Hutten, M. M. R., & Van der Lee, M. L. (2017). Effectiveness of two web-based interventions for chronic cancer-related fatigue compared to an active control condition: Results of the "Fitter na kanker" randomized controlled trial. *Journal of Medical Internet Research, 19,* e336.

30. Reynolds, L. M., Bissett, I. P., Porter, D., & Consedine, N. S. (2017). A brief mindfulness intervention is associated with negative outcomes in a randomised controlled trial among chemotherapy patients. *Mindfulness, 8,* 1291–1303.

31. Eisendrath, S. J., Gillung, E., Delucchi, K. L., Segal, Z. V., Nelson, J. C., McInnes, L. A., . . . Feldman, M. D. (2016). A randomized controlled trial of mindfulness-based cognitive therapy for treatment-resistant depression. *Psychotherapy and Psychosomatics, 85,* 99–110.

32. Goldin, P. R., Morrison, A., Jazaieri, H., Brozovich, F., Heimberg, R., & Gross, J. J. (2016). Group CBT versus MBSR for social anxiety disorder: A randomized controlled trial. *Journal of Consulting and Clinical Psychology, 5,* 427–437.

33. Meyers, L., Vollner, E. K., McCallum, E. B., Thuras, P., Shallcross, S., Velasquez, T., & Meis, L. (2017). Treating veterans with PTSD and borderline personality symptoms in a 12-week intensive outpatient setting: Findings from a pilot program. *Journal of Traumatic Stress, 30,* 178–181.

34. Kristeller, J., Wolever, R. Q., & Sheets, V. (2014). Mindfulness-based eating awareness training (MB-EAT) for binge eating: A randomized clinical trial. *Mindfulness, 5,* 282–297.

35. Chiesa, A., & Serretti, A. (2014). Are mindfulness-based interventions effective for substance use disorders? A systematic review of the evidence. *Substance Use and Misuse, 49,* 492–512.

36. Khoury, B., Lecomte, T., Fortin, G., Masse, M., Therien, V. B., Chapleu, M. A., . . . Hofmann, S. G. (2013). Mindfulness-based therapy: Comprehensive meta-analysis. *Clinical Psychology Review, 33,* 763–771.

37. Öst, L. G. (2008). Efficacy of the third wave of behavioral therapies: A systematic review and meta-analysis. *Behaviour Research and Therapy, 46,* 296–321.

38. Teasdale, J. D., Segal, Z. V., Williams, J. M., Ridgeway, V. A., Soulsby, J. M., & Lau, M. A. (2000). Prevention of relapse/recurrence in major depression by mindfulness-based cognitive therapy. *Journal of Consulting and Clinical Psychology, 68,* 615–623.

39. Williams, J. M. G., Crane, C., Barnhofer, T., Brennan, K., Duggan, D. S., Fennell, M. J. V., . . . Russell, I. T. (2014). Mindfulness-based cognitive therapy for preventing relapse in recurrent depression: A randomized dismantling trial. *Journal of Consulting and Clinical Psychology, 82,* 275–286.

40. Kuyken, W., Hayes, R., Barrett, B., Byng, R., Dalgleish, T., Kessler, D., . . . Byford, S. (2015). Effectiveness and cost-effectiveness of mindfulness-based cognitive therapy compared with maintenance antidepressant treatment in the prevention of depressive relapse or recurrence (PREVENT): A randomised controlled trial. *The Lancet, 386,* 63–73.

41. Chiesa, A., Castagner, V., Andrisano, C., Serretti, A., Mandelli, L., Porcelli, S., & Giommi, F. (2015). Mindfulness-based cognitive therapy vs. psychoeducation for patients with major depression who did not achieve remission following antidepressant treatment. *Psychiatry Research, 226,* 474–483.

42. Kabat-Zinn, J., Massion, A. O., Kristeller, J., Peterson, L. G., Fletcher, K. E., Pbert, L., . . . Santorelli, S. F. (1992). Effectiveness of a meditation-based stress reduction program in the treatment of anxiety disorders. *American Journal of Psychiatry, 149,* 936–943.

43. Koszycki, D., Benger, M., Shlik, J., & Bradwejn, J. (2007). Randomized trial of a meditation-based stress reduction program and cognitive behavior therapy in generalized social anxiety disorder. *Behaviour Research and Therapy, 45,* 2518–2526.

44. American Psychiatric Association. (2013). *Diagnostic and statistical manual of mental disorders* (5th ed.). Washington, DC: American Psychiatric Publishing.

45. Lineham, M. M. (1993). *Cognitive-behavioral treatment of borderline personality disorder.* New York: Guilford Press.

46. Stoffers-Winterling, J. M., Völlm, B. A., Rücker, G., Timmer, A., Huband, N., & Lieb, K. (2012). Psychological therapies for people with borderline personality disorder. *Cochrane Database of Systematic Reviews, 8,* Article ID: CD005652. doi:10.1002/14651858.CD005652.pub2

47. Marzal, M., & Górska, D. (2015). The regulative function of mentalization and mindfulness in borderline personality organization. *Current Issues in Personality Psychology, 3,* 51–63.

48. Panos, P. T., Jackson, J. W., Hasan, O., & Panos, A. (2014). Meta-analysis and systematic review assessing the efficacy of dialectical behavior therapy (DBT). *Research on Social Work Practice, 24,* 213–223.

49. U.S. Department of Veteran Affairs (2017, September 15). *VA Releases Veteran Suicide Statistics by State.* Retrieved on March 12, 2018, from https://www.va.gov/opa/pressrel/pressrelease.cfm?id=2951

50. Keenan, K., Hipwell, A., Feng, X., Babinski, D., Hinze, A., Rischall, M., & Henneberger, A. (2008). Subthreshold symptoms of depression in preadolescent girls are stable and predictive of depressive disorders. *Journal of the American Academy of Child and Adolescent Psychiatry, 47,* 1433–1442.

51. Greenberg, M. T., & Harris, A. R. (2012). Nurturing mindfulness in children and youth: Current state of research. *Child Development Perspectives, 6,* 161–166.

52. Britton, W. B., Lepp, N. E., Niles, H. F., Rocha, T., Fisher, N. E., & Gold, J. S. (2014). A randomized controlled pilot trial of classroom-based mindfulness meditation compared to an active control condition in sixth-grade children. *Journal of School Psychology, 52,* 263–278.

53. Mendelson, T., Greenberg, M. T., Dariotis, J. K., Gould, L. F., Rhoades, B. L., & Leaf, P. J. (2010). Feasibility and preliminary outcomes of a school-based mindfulness intervention for urban youth. *Journal of Abnormal Child Psychology, 38,* 985–994.

54. Zoogman, S., Goldberg, S. B., Hoyt, W. T., & Miller, L. (2015). Mindfulness interventions with youth: A meta-analysis. *Mindfulness, 6,* 290–302.

55. Bamber, M. D., & Schneider, J. K. (2016). Mindfulness-based meditation to decrease stress and anxiety in college students: A narrative synthesis of the research. *Educational Research Review, 18,* 1–32.

56. Khoury, B., Sharma, M., Rush, S. E., & Fournier, C. (2015). Mindfulness-based stress reduction for healthy individuals: A meta-analysis. *Journal of Psychosomatic Research, 78,* 519–528.

57. Barnes, S., Brown, K. W., Krusemark, E., Campbell, W. K., & Rogge, R. D. (2007). The role of mindfulness in romantic relationship satisfaction and responses to relationship stress. *Journal of Marital and Family Therapy, 33,* 482–500.

58. Carson, J. W., Carson, K. M., Gil, K. M., & Baucom, D. H. (2004). Mindfulness-based relationship enhancement. *Behavior Therapy, 35,* 471–494.

59. Wachs, K., & Cordova, J. V. (2007). Mindful relating: Exploring mindfulness and emotion repertoires in intimate relationships. *Journal of Marital and Family Therapy, 33,* 464–481.

60. Adair, K. C., Boulton, A. J., & Algoe, S. B. (2017). The effect of mindfulness on relationship satisfaction via perceived responsiveness: Findings from a dyadic study of heterosexual partners. *Mindfulness,* Advance online publication. doi:10.1007/s12671-017-0801-3

61. Baer, R. A., Smith, G. T., Hopkins, J., Krietemeyer, J., & Toney, L. (2006). Using self-report assessment methods to explore facets of mindfulness. *Assessment, 13,* 27–45.

62. Carson, J. W., Carson, K. M., Gil, K. M., & Baucom, D. H. (2007). Self-expansion as a mediator of relationship improvements in a mindfulness intervention. *Journal of Marital and Family Therapy, 33,* 517–528.

63. Atkinson, B. (2015). Mindfulness and the skillful navigation of relationship. *Familiendynamik: Systemische Praxis und Forschung, 40,* 106–120.

64. Shapiro, S. L., & Schwartz, G. E. (1999). Intentional systemic mindfulness: An integrative model for self-regulation and health. *Advances in Mind-Body Medicine, 15,* 128–134.

65. World Health Organization. (1946). *Constitution of the World Health Organization.* Retrieved on March 12, 2018, from http://www.who.int/governance/eb /who_constitution_en.pdf

CHAPTER FOUR

Evidence-Based Portable Mindful Strategies for Well-Being

Luc R. Pelletier and Jill E. Bormann

In our hectic, information-drenched realities, individuals seek a state of well-being. Although there are a number of maladaptive ways of coping (alcohol, drugs, and self-abusive behavior), many individuals look toward formal and informal religions and spiritual practices to cope with everyday challenges. For those with advanced or enduring illness, the search for comfort also includes a search for meaning and purpose to alleviate distress. For example, 84 percent of cancer patients relied on religion or spiritual beliefs as ways to cope with illness and its physical and emotional effects;[1] 72 percent of these patients believed that their spiritual needs were being met minimally or not at all by the medical establishment.[2] Thus, in addition to medical regimens, other religious and spiritual interventions need to be accessible to help people cope. Mantram repetition (MR), slowing down, and one-pointed attention are effective, evidence-based coping interventions. Together they make up what is called the mantram repetition program (MRP)—a set of personal, portable skills for calming the mind, body, and spirit. This program was originally taught in an eight-week (90 minutes per week) group format but has also been delivered individually, using a variety of webinar formats, and has been adapted for situations where there are few or limited resources for meetings.

The health reform imperative has emphasized the need to move from treating the illness (medical and clinical needs) to treating the whole person.[3] This derives from consumers empowered to be more engaged in their treatment. More engaged and activated patients experience better quality care at lower costs.[4,5] Whole health encompasses physical as well as emotional (including spiritual) well-being.

The Stress Response and Retraining the Mind

In stress-response studies since the 1930s, researchers have studied the body's unique ability to balance itself through the peripheral nervous system, which serves to arouse (take action; fight/flight) or inhibit response (rest). Stress activates arousal, and our natural inclination, through conditioning, is to react. MR helps slow down one's thinking and focus one's attention. MR provides a "short pause," putting enough space between the triggering event and the individual's reaction to enable him or her to choose *how or whether to respond* to a stressful situation (see Figure 4.1).

Choosing and Using a Mantram

The first step in employing MR is choosing a mantram. Easwaran proposed that "the mantram is a short, powerful spiritual formula for the highest power that we can conceive of—whether we call it God, or the ultimate reality, or the self within. Whatever name we call it, we are calling up what is best and deepest in ourselves."[6] A list of recommended mantrams can be found in Table 4.1. Mantrams recommended by Easwaran are marked with an asterisk.

The mantram can be repeated anytime, anywhere. The mantram can be spoken silently or out loud or it can be written repeatedly. It can be used while waiting, to redirect wandering attention; while walking or exercising; before, during, or after meals; to manage emotions such as depression, fear, frustration, or anxiety; and before sleep or upon awakening. There are three progressive stages of mantram practice: mechanical, experiential, and habitual. Mechanical is the first stage of just repeating the mantram in a rote way—it is monotonous and seemingly has little effect at first. This repetition

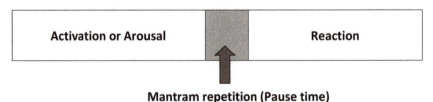

Mantram repetition (Pause time)

Figure 4.1   Reducing Reactivity through Mantram Repetition

Table 4.1   Choosing Your Mantram

If you have this in mind...	Then choose this mantram...
Christian	
St. Francis of Assisi's phrase	My God and My All or Deus meus et omnia*
Lord of the Heart (Aramaic)	Maranatha (Mah-rah-nah-tha)
Lord have mercy	Kyrie Eleison or Gospodi pomilui* (Kir-ee-ay Ee-lay-ee-sone)
Christ have mercy	Christe Eleison (Kreest-ay Ee-lay-ee-sone)
Son of God	Jesus, Jesus*
Mother of Jesus	Hail Mary or Ave Maria*
Jesus Prayer	Lord Jesus Christ son of God, have mercy on me* or Om Yesu Christu*
Hindu	
Eternal joy within (Gandhi's mantram)	Rama, Rama* (Rah-mah)
	Hare Rama, Hare Krishna
Invocation to beauty and fearlessness	Om Namah Shivaya* (Ohm Nah-mah Shee-vah-yah)
A call for universal love	Om Prema (Ohm Pray-Mah)
Invocation to eternal peace	Om Shanti (Ohm Shawn-tee)
I am that self within	So Ham (So hum)
	Om Sri Ram, jai Ram, jai jai Ram*
In honor of the Divine Mother	Om Bhavani*
Buddhist	
The jewel (the Self) is in the lotus of the heart	Om ManePadme Hum* (Ohm mah-nee pod-may-hume)
I bow to the Buddha of Infinite Light	Namo Amida Butsu* (Na-mo ah-mee-dah boot-soo)
I bow to the Buddha	Namo Butsaya (naw-moh boot-sie-yah)
Judaic	
Peace, completeness	Shalom (Shah-lome)
Blessed art Thou, King of the Universe	Barukh Atah Adonoi* (Bah-rookh At-tah Ah-doh-nigh)
Lord of the Universe	Ribono Shel Olam* (Ree-boh-no Shel O-lahm)

(continued)

Table 4.1   *(continued)*

Native American	
Great Spirit	O Wakan Tanka (Oh Wah-Kahn Tahn-Kah)
Islamic/Arabic/Muslim	
Lord God, the One	Allah, Allah* (Alla)
God is Great	Allah Akbar (Alla-Okbar)
In the name of God, the merciful, the compassionate	Bismallah ir-Rahman ir-Rahim* (Beese-mah-lah ir-Rah-mun ir-Rah-heem)

*Recommended by Eknath Easwaran.

is necessary, however, for the second stage—experiential—which is a period of self-awareness. In this stage, there is increased awareness of one's thought processes, and when repeating a mantram, one "experiences the pause." There is a conscious change in reactivity. Finally, the third stage is habitual, which comes over a long period of time. The goal is for mantram practice to become an automatic habit with positive, stress-relieving benefits.

Slowing Down

> If you let cloudy water settle, it will become clear. If you let your upset mind settle, your course will also become clear.
>
> —Gautama Buddha[7]

Slowing down. This term is antithetical to all that we were taught in our formation—at school and in our workplaces: hurry, hurry, hurry. It doesn't comport to the fast-paced, stimuli-rich, constant motion that is part of our everyday lives, but slowing down is a critical portable strategy for well-being. In our hectic pace, the natural pause has been removed from our lives. Consider the progression of various tools and technologies over the past decades. These innovations typically involved cutting time, making things faster. For example, buttons became zippers, which became Velcro. People used stoves, then pressure cookers, and now microwaves. Washboards were replaced with the wringer/washer; now people use washers and dryers. People once used an abacus, then an adding machine, now a calculator. Desktop computers were replaced with laptop computers; now people use their smartphones or tablets.

In this speeded-up world, our thoughts and actions are frantic. To determine if you are going too fast, complete the adapted survey originally developed by *A Business Management Daily*[8] (see Table 4.2). If you have concluded that you are moving at too quick a pace and want to slow down, use the

Table 4.2   10 Reasons You May Need a Pause

Read the following statement and give yourself:

- 2 points for each statement that *fits you perfectly*;
- 1 point for each that *fits you somewhat*;
- 0 points for each one that *doesn't sound like you at all*.

Then review the table at the end to score how fast you are going:

	Circle Your Score		
1. I always eat quickly.	0	1	2
2. I talk rapidly.	0	1	2
3. I often finish people's sentences.	0	1	2
4. I almost always feel pressed for time.	0	1	2
5. I often feel pressured at work.	0	1	2
6. I can feel my blood pressure climb in slow checkout lines.	0	1	2
7. I follow the car in front of me closely when driving.	0	1	2
8. I often do two or more things at once to save time.	0	1	2
9. I feel as if I'm wasting time if I do only one thing at a time.	0	1	2
10. I get restless if I have to sit still.	0	1	2
Total			

SCORING:	
11 to 20:	Your fast ways are very well could be compromising your health, your well-being and your career.
6 to 10:	You're moving fast. You'd enjoy life more if you slow down and take a pause.
0 to 5:	Good for you! You're taking life at a reasonable pace!

Source: Adapted from *A Business Management Daily*, 2017.

survey to reshape your priorities and time. For example, pick an item on the list (e.g., *I always eat fast*), and consider the following:

1. Plan ahead when you will eat during the day.
2. Prior to eating, repeat your mantram, put your phone and tasks aside, and become aware of any physical hunger and preferences for food and drink.
3. Acknowledge that this time is only for eating with a specific intention to satisfy your body's physiological needs.

4. Decide if you will be alone or with others during the meal. Avoid looking at the phone, TV, or computer.

5. Be mindful of the taste of the food, the texture, and the smells. Notice how you are feeling.

6. If you get distracted or start speeding up, acknowledge the distraction, briefly repeat your mantram, slow down, and bring your attention back to eating/drinking.

7. Be grateful that you have food and drink that replenishes your body and promotes physical and emotional resilience.

Developing One-Pointed Attention

One-pointed attention is the opposite of multitasking. When we "mono-task," our full attention is on one activity. By practicing mantram repetition, we are practicing one-pointed attention on the mantram. By doing so, we increase our ability to focus on other tasks at will. There are advantages to monotasking or one-pointed attention:

- increased efficiency
- fewer mistakes and rework (or waste)
- increased mental calmness in achieving one goal at a time
- increased quality of work
- less stress overall

The brain is limited in its ability to attend. Easwaran proposes six ways to tame an unruly mind:

1. Start with meditation.
2. Do only one thing at a time.
3. Listen.
4. Know where to put your attention.
5. Learn to drop work at will.
6. Keep your attention in the present.[9]

Several one-pointed attention exercises are provided below. Try them or develop some of your own.

In relationships: Practice giving your complete attention to the person you are talking to or who is talking to you. Try to listen without thinking of what you are going to say next. When faced with an interruption or distraction, give *more* attention to the person you are with.

During meal time: Give your entire attention to eating and tasting your food. Turn off the radio, TV, or other background noise. Notice what happens when you really taste what you are eating.

When procrastinating: Practice one-pointed attention on a task you have neglected or postponed for a long time (such as cleaning the closet or drawers). Choose something that you find difficult or distasteful, and give your entire attention to it. Set a timer, and tell yourself you can quit after half an hour unless you find yourself involved in the task.

With challenging projects: Choose a difficult project, and bring your complete attention to it for a predetermined period of time. Notice how your mind will try to distract you, but bring your attention back over and over until your time is up.

While driving or riding: Give your attention to the act of driving a car. Turn off the radio or music. If you are a passenger on the bus, give your attention to the act of riding or looking out the window.

In the workplace: Give your attention to each task you are doing (even if for only a split second), whether it is talking on the phone with patients or with colleagues, researching a project, answering e-mails, or filing documents.

The MRP has been shown through randomized clinical trials, one-group and mixed-methods intervention studies, qualitative interview studies, and real-world studies to significantly affect posttraumatic symptoms, psychological distress, and quality of life. These portable interventions are effective with a wide array of populations.

Types of Populations and Research Outcomes of the MRP

There is a growing body of research evidence supporting some positive health benefits of the MRP. The first studies on the MRP were conducted in groups of veterans with a variety of chronic illnesses, such as diabetes, heart disease, respiratory problems, and painful conditions.[10, 11] These preliminary studies did not include any control or comparison groups, but outcomes clearly indicated significant reductions in self-reported perceived stress, anxiety, and anger along with improvements in quality of life and spiritual well-being.[12] Interviews with veterans confirmed these findings. Here is a quote from a veteran MRP participant about how the mantram helped manage symptoms of insomnia: "On days I don't use my sleep medication . . . those are the days when I use my mantram and that's when I wake up at night, and I know that I shouldn't be waking up because of work, you know, intensely, I work long hours and so . . . I will use the mantram [for insomnia] and it works."

The first large randomized controlled trial of the MRP was conducted in adults living with HIV/AIDS. The program was compared to an active educational control group where both arms of the study received social support in a group setting. Although there were significant reductions in perceived stress and anxiety in both groups, the most significant finding from the MRP participants was a reduction in levels of anger.[13] This improvement remained consistent at two-month follow-up. In addition, there was evidence that greater frequency of mantram practice was associated with improvements in quality of life and spiritual well-being. In other words, those who repeated their mantrams the most (highest users) demonstrated a greater sense of spiritual faith/assurance (i.e., belief that everything will be okay) than the moderate users. And both high and moderate mantram users had better health outcomes than the control group (those without a mantram).[14]

Health-care employees are continually coping with burnout and compassion fatigue in caring for patients in very stressful, and sometimes even hostile or violent, work environments. In a clinical trial of nurse managers in South Korea, findings indicated improvements in spiritual well-being, spiritual integrity, and leadership practice.[15] A study of health-care providers showed that participation in the MRP resulted in lower levels of stress, anger, and anxiety, and also improvements in quality of life and spiritual well-being.[16] In another study testing a Web-based version of the MRP targeting health-care providers for stress and burnout, findings demonstrated lower levels of exhaustion—a characteristic of burnout.[17] In addition, the majority of health-care providers reported practicing slowing down and one-pointed attention in the workplace up to two months afterward. One example of a health-care provider's mantram use was more personal with regard to a memory of a coworker who died: "The reason why that situation [coworker's death] prompted me to use my mantram was because every night as I would leave my job, I would actually go past this one particular location where my coworker would be, as if he was pondering or thinking . . . and now when I reach that spot every day, I think about him and more so, I think I reverse the situation and I put myself in his place and so I use the mantram to kind of take me away from that space . . . that mental space and to refocus on what I'm supposed to be doing."

Not only health-care providers but also family caregivers of veterans with dementia have found ways to use mantram repetition to help them with the burden of caregiving.[18] For example, when family caregivers were asked about situations where they used MR, one responded: "Um, well, financial situations, like my mother is ill right now, so having to help her dealing with dementia; so my sisters and I and my dad are having to deal with taking care of her, worrying about her constantly, and then my dad's health isn't great either, but better than she is, you know. Just anything, the phone rings—it's like, I hope it's not something wrong, so those kind of situations." In this circumstance, hearing the phone ring had triggered the fear of bad news, and repeating a mantram interrupted that fear and perhaps prevented the possibility of catastrophizing.

Another example of MR for managing caregiver stress illustrates how MR can provide "something to do" when a caregiver feels helpless. This quote also demonstrates how the practice of MR can become automatic with prolonged, intentional use over time. "Well, dealing with my mom with her dementia, you know, sitting there. She doesn't respond, but she just sits there and you know, it's very stressful and it's almost scary because, you know, there she is, your mother, and she doesn't know you and doesn't respond and then, so you start worrying and stressing out about it, you know. I find myself sitting there repeating the mantram so I can calm myself down from stressing over, you know. There's not a whole lot I can do, but the mantram, it's automatically triggering on its own."

Veterans with posttraumatic stress disorder (PTSD) have reported numerous ways and situations where repeating a mantram has helped them manage symptoms of hyperarousal, avoidance, and flashbacks. Some examples include nightmares and reexperiencing traumatic events.[19] "I use mantram at night so I will sleep the night. I have nightmares from Vietnam and it wakes me up. So I start my mantram and it calms me down and I just keep doing it and I fall asleep, you know, with the mantram being repeated over and over and over." Another veteran stated: "I was falling asleep on the couch watching the news and a helicopter went overhead and it was circling around out on the street here and I found myself dealing with some of the problems in Vietnam . . . I turned everything off and just sat there in the dark and repeated the mantram to calm myself down while that helicopter was flying overhead. It worked pretty good. It calmed me down and it wasn't that I was scared or anything, but that it was kind of like, um, the memories of what a helicopter overhead sounds like. It [mantram] relaxes me and calms me down."

In response to a question about how he used mantram for dealing with a trauma-related flashback/incident, a veteran replied: "[Mantram repetition results in] more of a calming sensation than anything else. It [mantram repetition] took the edge off of the feelings that I had about the incident and caused me to reflect on it more and it kind of saved me from a heart attack, that situation, really. You can get, you know, so tied into these things to where they build up and build up and build up and the mantram helps me take the edge off of it and wipe the situation back down so it's not as disturbing to my system, not only emotionally, but physically, as well." In this example, repeating a mantram does not entirely dispel one's emotional discomfort or negative feelings but provides the ability to take the edge off those uncomfortable feelings, thus making them more manageable.

In another real-world multisite study, veterans reported significant improvements in symptoms of depression, anxiety, and somatization.[20] In addition, they experienced increased levels of spiritual well-being as characterized by a greater sense of meaning and purpose, increased peacefulness, and higher levels of faith/assurance.[21] In essence, veterans with PTSD reported that MR helped them calm down whenever they felt anxiety, impatience, frustration, or irritability.

MRP has also been taught to underserved, vulnerable populations, such as homeless women. In a pilot study, a condensed form of the MRP (provided within a two-hour session) was taught to a community sample of homeless women (*n* = 29) with a focus on insomnia.[22] The women were taught how to choose and use a mantram and then were given small laminated cards that were easy to carry and served as a reminder to practice repeating the mantram during the day, every day, and also at night before sleep. After one week of practice, the majority reported improvements in insomnia, thus demonstrating the simplicity and low cost of the program as well as its potential for wider dissemination among a variety of populations.

Summary

MR, slowing down, and one-pointed attention are portable spiritual tools that individuals can use to retrain the mind. They work synergistically to provide a pause in our hectic lives. Through habitual use, these simple, no-cost tools can help alleviate stress. In his book *The Art of Stillness*, Iyer concludes: "In an age of speed, I began to think, nothing could be more invigorating than going slow. In an age of distraction, nothing could feel more luxurious than paying attention. And in an age of constant movement, nothing is more urgent than sitting still."[23]

These mindfulness strategies have been found to be effective in reducing a variety of symptoms in various populations.

References

1. Vallurupalli, M., Lauderdale, K., Balboni, M. J., Phelps, A. C., Kachnic, L. A., VanderWeele, T. J., & Balboni, T. A. (2012). The role of spirituality and religious coping in the quality of life of patients with advanced cancer receiving palliative radiation therapy. *Journal of Supportive Oncology, 10*(2), 81–87.

2. Balboni, T. A., Vanderwerker, L. C., Block, S. D., Paulk, M. E., Lathan, C. S., Peteet, J. R., & Prigerson, H. G. (2007). Religiousness and spiritual support among advanced cancer patients and associations with end-of-life treatment preferences and quality of life. *Journal of Clinical Oncology, 25*(5), 555–560.

3. National Quality Forum. (2016). *Issue brief: Strategies for change: A collaborative journey to transform advanced illness care*. Washington, DC: Author.

4. Pelletier, L. R., & Stichler, J. F. (2013). Action brief: Patient engagement and activation: A health care reform imperative and improvement opportunity for nursing. *Nursing Outlook, 61*(1), 51–54.

5. Rickert, J. (2012, January 24). Patient-centered care: What it means and how to get there. *Health Affairs Blog*. Retrieved on March 12, 2018, from http://healthaffairs.org/blog/2012/01/24/patient-centered-care-what-it-means-and-how-to-get-there/

6. Easwaran, E. (2013). The power of mantram. *Blue Mountain: A Journal for Spiritual Living, 24*(3), 1–4.

7. Kornfield, J. (1994). *Buddha's little instruction book.* New York: Bantam Books.

8. A Business Management Daily. (2017, August 21). Do you need more "think time" in your day? A 16-question self-quiz. *A Business Management Daily.* Retrieved on March 12, 2018, from https://www.businessmanagementdaily .com/1681/do-you-need-more-think-time-in-your-day-a-16-question-self-quiz

9. Easwaran, E. (2014). Six ways to tame an unruly mind. *Blue Mountain Journal, 25*(2), 11–22.

10. Bormann, J. E., Gifford, A. L., Shively, M., Smith, T. L., Redwine, L., Kelly, A., . . . Belding, W. (2006). Effects of spiritual mantram repetition on HIV outcomes: A randomized controlled trial. *Journal of Behavioral Medicine, 29*(4), 359–376.

11. Bormann, J. E., Smith, T. L., Becker, S., Gershwin, M., Pada, L., Grudsinski, A. H., & Nurmi, E. A. (2005). Efficacy of frequent mantram repetition on stress, quality of life, and spiritual well-being in veterans: A pilot study. *Journal of Holistic Nursing, 23*(4), 395–414.

12. Bormann, J. E., Smith, T. L., Becker, S., Gershwin, M., Pada, L., Grudsinski, A. H., & Nurmi, E. A. (2005). Efficacy of frequent mantram repetition on stress, quality of life, and spiritual well-being in veterans: A pilot study. *Journal of Holistic Nursing, 23*(4), 395–414.

13. Bormann, J. E., Gifford, A. L., Shively, M., Smith, T. L., Redwine, L., Kelly, A., & Belding, W. (2006). Effects of spiritual mantram repetition on HIV outcomes: A randomized controlled trial. *Journal of Behavioral Medicine, 29*(4), 359–376.

14. Bormann, J. E., Gifford, A. L., Shively, M., Smith, T. L., Redwine, L., Kelly, A., & Belding, W. (2006). Effects of spiritual mantram repetition on HIV outcomes: A randomized controlled trial. *Journal of Behavioral Medicine, 29*(4), 359–376.

15. Yong, J., Kim, J., Park, J., Seo, I., & Swinton, J. (2011). Effects of spirituality training program on the spiritual and psychosocial well-being of hospital middle manager nurses in Korea. *Journal of Continuing Education in Nursing, 42*(6), 280–288.

16. Bormann, J. E., Becker, S., Gershwin, M., Kelly, A., Pada, L., Smith, T. L., & Gifford, A. L. (2006). Relationship of frequent mantram repetition to emotional and spiritual well-being in healthcare workers. *Journal of Continuing Education in Nursing, 37*(5), 218–224.

17. Bormann, J. E., Walter, K. H., Leary, S., & Glaser, D. (2017). An internet-delivered mantram repetition program for spiritual well-being and mindfulness for health care workers. *Spirituality in Clinical Practice, 4*, 64–73.

18. Bormann, J. E., Warren, K. A., Regalbuto, L., Glaser, D., Kelly, A., Schnack, J., & Hinton, L. (2009). A spiritually-based caregiver intervention with telephone delivery for family caregivers of veterans with dementia. *Family and Community Health, 32*(4), 345–353.

19. Bormann, J. E., Hurst, S., & Kelly, A. (2013). Responses to mantram repetition program from veterans with posttraumatic stress disorder: A qualitative analysis. *Journal of Rehabilitation Research & Development, 50*(6), 769–784.

20. Buttner, M. M., Bormann, J. E., Weingart, K., Andrews, T., Ferguson, M., & Afari, N. (2016). Multi-site evaluation of a complementary, spiritually-based intervention for veterans: The mantram repetition program. *Complementary Therapy in Clinical Practice, 22,* 74–79. doi:10.1016/j.clcp.2015.12.008

21. Buttner, M. M., Bormann, J. E., Weingart, K., Andrews, T., Ferguson, M., & Afari, N. (2016). Multi-site evaluation of a complementary, spiritually-based intervention for veterans: The mantram repetition program. *Complementary Therapy in Clinical Practice, 22,* 74–79. doi:10.1016/j.clcp.2015.12.008

22. Weinrich, S. P., Bormann, J. E., Glaser, D., Hardin, S., Barger, M., Lizarrage, C., Del Rio, J., & Allard, C. B. (2016). Mantram repetition with homeless women: A pilot study. *Holistic Nursing Practice, 30*(6), 360–367. doi:10.1097/HNP.0000000000000138

23. Iyer, P. (2014). *The art of stillness: Adventures in going nowhere.* New York: Simon & Schuster.

CHAPTER FIVE

Spiritual Surrender: A Paradoxical Means of Empowered Coping with Illness while Discovering Transcendent Meaning and Purpose in Life

Kathleen Wall, Sandra Velasco-Scott, and Arielle Warner

Spiritual surrender is not a passive act. It is an active giving over of self-protection and self-will, a vote of confidence in the Infinite, a decision to trust. It is releasing the erroneous idea of a separate self. . . . Living a surrendered life requires practice and daily commitment.
—Yogacharya Ellen Grace O'Brian, *Living for the Sake of the Soul*[1]

Most religious and spiritual traditions include spiritual surrender as a means of transcending human suffering. Surrender is a multifaceted transformative experience that includes reevaluating meanings and actualizing a higher life purpose. Research indicates that the practice of spiritual surrender can paradoxically empower people and provide them with enhanced meaning and improved well-being when facing uncontrollable circumstances like serious illnesses. Effective surrender is not to be understood as a passive giving up but rather as an active partnering with a personalized sense of the Divine. Positive health effects have been found with active collaborative surrender versus other religious/spiritual practices of coping (e.g., passive deferment—handing everything over to a higher power—or pleading for a self-determined outcome).[2] This is especially true for people coping with circumstances over which they can exert little control, such as multiple health issues (e.g., hospitalized medical patients with multiple diagnoses).[3]

Research on spirituality in coping with illness attempted to answer questions regarding the effects of using different types of religious/spiritual coping. Within this research, Cole and Pargament[2] differentiated five types of religious coping, including spiritual surrender:

1. *Self-directing:* People using the self-directing approach understand themselves as the locus of decision-making control. They may or may not have a spiritual belief system.

2. *Collaborative:* The collaborative coping style is a partnership between the individual and a transcendent power.

3. *Deferring:* People abandon personal responsibility, and the entire situation is resolved by willfully following the tenets of individuals' religious/spiritual beliefs.

4. *Pleading:* Individuals use a pleading style to petition God for a self-directed outcome such as a cure. They fail to recognize a potential outcome that would be for the greater good.

5. *Spiritual surrender:* The individual implements solutions to problems and collaborates with a transcendent power to develop a sense of coherence and meaning while apprehending a higher life purpose in difficult circumstances.

Studies on coping styles show varying degrees of beneficial outcomes. However, Cole and Pargament's research suggests that the collaborative approach is linked with better outcomes than the deferring,[4] self-directing,[5] or pleading[6] approaches. These results were consistent in situations like severe illness where stress is extreme and personal control is diminished. In serious illness, researchers found increased depression in people using the self-directing approach, while depression decreased in individuals using collaborative approaches.[2] Most favorable health and psycho-social-spiritual well-being outcomes have been found with collaborative coping styles, which is the definition of spiritual surrender: "aligning one's personal will with the Divine will."

In this chapter, we distinguish spiritual surrender as an alternative means of coping with illness, and we present the qualities of spiritual surrender. These qualities are then described by the surrender experiences of cancer survivors participating in Psycho-Spiritual Integrative Therapy (PSIT). Research on the health effects of spiritual surrender are presented, including spiritual/ religious coping styles, transcendent meaning-making processes, and counseling methods incorporating spiritual surrender for people enduring physical illness. We describe how PSIT incorporates multiple spiritual practices as a developmental process culminating in spiritual surrender and a capacity to live one's highest life purpose with enhanced well-being.

Qualities of Spiritual Surrender

Spiritual surrender is not to be confused with concepts of defeat or with other spiritual coping styles, such as deferring all responsibility to God or pleading with God for a personally desired outcome. Surrender is a distinct form of spiritual coping with illness and an elevating spiritual practice that can result in an expanded sense of self and life purpose. It is "an inner shift from a personal to transpersonal . . . state of consciousness" (p. 106).[7] According to integral yoga (Vedic) cosmology as described by Sri Aurobindo,[8] "[Surrender] is a collaborative process of actively accepting one's personal sense of the Sacred, and going through a progressive self-giving experience to the Divine, within one's self, in full trust and complete confidence, regardless of what might occur in life" (pp. 586–587).

Cole and Pargament[2] describe spiritual surrender as not simply a coping mechanism but as a profound spiritual discipline within multiple spiritual traditions performed in times of difficulty and as a continuous practice. Surrender may help in the process of making meaning of life, since it involves the recognition of a higher value, a broader perspective of a greater good, a higher spiritual life purpose, and a transcendent higher power even in seemingly negative situations.

One quality of spiritual surrender is "self-transcendence."[2] The individual sees him- or herself in a relationship with a higher power or transcendent reality and not as the center of the world. Consequently, the individual does not search for personal control over a situation but relinquishes control to a greater transcendent reality. This shift from control to transcendence is referred to as a transformation of significance wherein there is a reappraisal of one's thoughts and behaviors from identifying with personal control to connection with the transpersonal sacred. Spiritual surrender is a multifaceted shift in motivation, perceptions, thought patterns, behaviors, emotions, and values. An expansive sense of self embraces a larger existence, releasing or setting aside personal desires for the sake of a greater good or existence, which can be described as commitment to spiritual beliefs and a higher aspirational life purpose. The subjective experience following surrender is characterized by an enhanced state of being that includes total acceptance, resulting in feelings of completeness, serenity, gratitude, and compassion.[2]

Many of these qualities of spiritual surrender are found in the descriptions captured in Velasco-Scott's[9] qualitative research analysis of the spiritual surrender experiences of cancer survivors participating in PSIT groups. Examples are presented below. Pseudonyms were used to protect participants' privacy.

This particular account comes from Jan, a practicing Catholic, Filipina breast-cancer survivor in her early seventies. In her own words, Jan described her collaborative spiritual surrender: "My will *softened blended with God* [emphasis added]." This resulted in a multidimensional transformative experience: "My spirit soared, flowed into one as if water from different sources, fused, merged, into a funnel-like path forming one stream headed toward the same direction, only one direction . . . to the open sea." From there she willingly released personal control and recognized that there was a higher purpose to her life: "I have an inner knowing that I am not in charge . . . realizing that all is planned before we were here and *all will be as it needs to be, to fulfill something far greater* [emphasis added]."

Due to her surrender experience, Jan felt serenity, release, and freedom: "The physical body felt like it was opening up, feeling lighter as if a door was opening and letting the sun shine in. . . . My feelings were ones of freedom, release from a tightly tethered rope, blood circulating easier, freer, flowing; my thoughts were one of welcome, as if a familiar face, safe, love filled, light drenched, life giving, breath, space, goodness. My thoughts were: 'It's okay, you have permission to feel what you are feeling. I felt acknowledgement, validation, worth."

Jan's experience of surrender first happened when she was diagnosed with stage III breast cancer, and it was collaborative as she sought to accept and trust her connection with God. She did not petition God for a predetermined outcome: "Yes [I surrendered]; it's more of acceptance and trust especially after diagnosis. I didn't cry. I just asked to be held tight and for God to hold my hand every step of the way. Faith waivers, but this group program brings me more concrete ways to cope."

Difficulties surrendering were also dealt with by using spiritual practices incorporated into PSIT, including meditation, defining and encouraging collaborative spiritual surrender, and developing the ability to witness rather than overidentify with the body or mind: "I had been working on this these past weeks to help me stay present. When my mind slips to past, future, or running commentary, I tune in to my physical [body] response and immediately notice, close my eyes, a good knowledge of where the sensation is, how it is affecting my thoughts, then I focus deeper on the physical sensation, for example a knee or hip pain, a knot in my stomach. I take a deep breath to calm my thoughts, then smile or send the breath to that particular part to soften, soften, and melt away. The body awareness meditation has helped a lot, and then I think loving kindness to the body. I . . . 'witness' with my body as separate and then I avoid overidentification with it at that particular moment. I also have a 'mantra of surrender' which allows me to embrace all that is, and then I can let it go easier." However, softening and reframing the concept of surrender was helpful in dealing with this fear: "[Surrender] is frightening at times, but I need to soften the word to mean, perhaps acceptance, permission to let go, and consent to release to a higher power."

Jan's personal account of collaborative spiritual surrender beautifully exemplifies the qualities and multidimensional transcendent experience of surrender. In the next section, we explore what research tells us about how the qualities of spiritual surrender affect health and well-being when people are suffering from illness.

Research

Effects of Spiritual Surrender on Health and Well-Being

In this section, we focus on research concerning the health effects of spiritual surrender on people suffering from physical health conditions and related distress. Spiritual coping with addiction is addressed in this book (see chapter 16 by Sperry and Stoupas). The most direct evidence of the health effects of spiritual surrender come from research on coping with illness. In the research reviewed here, spiritual surrender is measured by self-reported scales. In some cases the scales also include other spiritual beliefs and practices. Findings are associative rather than direct causal relationships between spiritual surrender and health outcomes.

Clements and Ermakova[10] investigated the link between spiritual surrender and stress among 230 women with high-risk pregnancies. Surrender was measured through interviews using a surrender scale.[11] Stress was measured by a prenatal psychosocial profile that included actual and perceived stress. Women who reported that they were more surrendered had lower measured stress even when controlling for age, marital status, education, and number of children. The findings suggest that surrender and its associated lower stress levels could be explored as a mechanism by which spirituality influences health and could lead to interventions.

Pargament, Koenig, Tarakeshwar, and Hahn[12] conducted a longitudinal study of 268 medically ill elderly patients. They used the Religious Coping Scales (RCOPE), which includes the category *active religious surrender*, meaning an active giving up of control to God ("Did what I could and put the rest in God's hands"). In a two-year follow-up, active surrender significantly correlated with and predicted spiritual well-being outcomes and stress-related growth in the expected direction. No physical health measures significantly correlated with active surrender.

When controlling for relevant variables, the complete RCOPE Scales—covering multiple spiritual practices, such as active surrender, prayer, ritual, and attending church—demonstrate that religious coping was significantly predictive of spiritual outcomes and changes in mental and physical health. Generally, positive methods of religious coping (e.g., seeking spiritual support and belief in a benevolent God) were associated with improvements in health.[12] However, negative methods of religious coping (e.g., a punishing God's reappraisal and interpersonal religious discontent) were predictive of declines in health.[12] Patients who continued to struggle with religious/spiritual issues over time were also particularly at risk for health-related declines.

Those who were able to change negative practices to positive were not at greater health risk; however, those who persisted in negative religious/spiritual beliefs, such as believing in a punishing God/higher power and using coping practices such as deferring, were likely to decline in physical, mental, and spiritual health.[12] This last finding is an indication that people can change over time, and if they do resolve these transcendent meaning-making conflicts, they have better biopsychological-spiritual well-being. Similar results have been found in several studies of a spiritual meaning-making model of coping with illness,[13] which we review in the following section.

Research on the Health Effects of Spiritual Meaning Making

Illness sets off "a search for significance,"[2] a process to make meaning of life in the face of adversity. Park[13] posits a meaning-making model to explain the process. Two levels of meanings are identified: situational and global. Situational meanings are appraisals of the specific illness situation. Global meanings are general orienting systems, including sense of life purpose, self-identity, control, justice, and belief in God as well as larger goals and ideals of life. Global meanings are qualities of spiritual surrender. Park explains, "Spirituality can inform all aspects of global meaning, informing beliefs (e.g. nature of God and humanity, control, destiny, Karma) and providing ultimate motivation and primary goals for living and guidelines for achieving these goals, along with a deep sense of purpose and mattering" (p. 42).[13] Park recognizes multiple qualities of spiritual surrender in this statement, such as life purpose and idealized spiritual goals. Global spiritual meanings and associated qualities of surrender have been linked with health in multiple studies and are especially potent in serious illness.[13,14]

These multiple health benefits of meaning making are most salient when meanings are actually made (completed), which is called "meanings-made." Continually ruminating about the meanings can result in declining health.[15,16] "Meanings-made" results in experiences of qualities of spiritual surrender, such as feeling compassion, feeling a connection with the Divine, apprehending one's spiritual life purpose, and living a more spiritually oriented life.

Less commonly, "meanings-made" can result in a diminished spiritual life.[17] As presented in the coping research above, chronically fixed negative meanings, such as belief in a punishing God, have been linked to declining health, but not when people were able to transform and adopt positive spiritual meanings and practices.[12] Counselors and clergy may help people working through spiritual meaning making to address spiritual struggles and develop positive spiritual/religious coping practices, like collaborative spiritual surrender.

Using spiritual coping during an illness can result in growth and positive benefits, otherwise known as posttraumatic growth. Transformation arising from suffering is common in many religions, including Judaism, Buddhism, and Christianity. Spiritual coping methods are among the most robust and consistent predictors of reported growth.[18] For instance, in spiritual surrender, one might see collaboration with God's will as taking personal responsibility for switching to a healthy lifestyle. However, unresolved meaning making may lead to unhealthy behaviors, such as substance abuse. These unhealthy behaviors appear as a denial of personal responsibility, which can masquerade as spiritual surrender while actually being a deferring coping style.

Coping and meaning-making research may be used to counsel people dealing with illness to cultivate coping styles and practices, such as collaborative spiritual surrender, that are potent enhancers of biopsychosocial-spiritual well-being. In this quest, Pargament's RCOPE and Surrender Scales[19] can help counselors differentiate the styles of coping, distinguish collaborative from the deferring and pleading styles, and encourage the use of positive spiritual/religious practices like spiritual surrender and the resolution of spiritual meanings. Counseling interventions that may be helpful to this end are addressed in the next section.

Research on the Health Effects of Counseling Interventions Integrating Spiritual Surrender

Though the connection between spirituality and health is fairly well established, few studies have examined interventions that include spiritual surrender. A study[20] of 13 HIV patients using a spiritual intervention that included surrender showed significant reductions in depression and spiritual struggle and increases in positive religious coping.

Cole and Pargament[21] developed a counseling intervention named Re-Creating Your Life (RCYL), which includes spiritual surrender. Cole[22] studied the use of RCYL with breast-cancer patients and found that pain severity and depression increased in women in no-treatment control conditions while remaining relatively stable for patients in RCYL intervention. Results of a study of RCYL with heart patients were not as favorable.[23] Heart patients in the cognitive-behavioral intervention showed a significant reduction in anxiety, while anxiety remained stable for those in RCYL. Patients in the no-treatment control condition increased in anxiety. Cole and Pargament[21] reanalyzed the results and found that, unlike the cancer patients, who had high levels of depression and distress, the heart patients were less distressed. They concluded that medical treatment with pacemakers or defibrillators treated the heart patients' symptoms. In comparison to the cancer patients, the heart patients were living normally. Cole and Pargament[21] indicated that RCYL might be most suited for people in high-stress situations where personal control is limited.

Psycho-Spiritual Integrative Therapy (PSIT), a counseling method that explicitly includes collaborative spiritual surrender, has a small body of research with cancer survivors. Two qualitative studies of the surrender experience of cancer survivors participating in PSIT help us to grasp the qualities of spiritual surrender. Rosequist and colleagues'[24] study describes the surrender experiences of 12 breast-cancer survivors, describing surrender as a type of active acceptance coping that has many positive health benefits. Velasco-Scott's[9] qualitative research on the experience of spiritual surrender yielded rich descriptions of surrender's qualities in 12 PSIT participants suffering from a variety of cancers. Examples of these personal accounts are represented in this chapter.

The quantitative research on PSIT reveals positive physical, psychological, and spiritual well-being changes among cancer survivors participating in PSIT groups. Johnson[25] studied qualities of spiritual surrender, including self-transcendence, spiritual well-being, and spiritual growth, to determine if these qualities mediated health outcomes. In a study of 31 cancer survivors participating in eight-week PSIT groups, he found that changes (change scores) of self-transcendence, spiritual well-being, and spiritual growth were significantly correlated with changes in functional health, stress, and mood disorders in the expected direction (i.e., those who increased in self-transcendence reported improved health and quality of life). He also investigated the mechanisms of change through a mediation study of these components of spiritual surrender. When cancer survivors changed the most on measures of overall spiritual well-being (a quality of surrender), this change accounted for all their changes in stress and mood disturbances and partially accounted for their changes in depression. No significant links with functional health were established. Measures of spiritual growth were not found to have a significant effect on well-being. Johnson found that changes in self-transcendence partially accounted for changes in the expected direction in functional and mental health. Self-transcendence is a quality of spiritual surrender, so we understand from these results that it significantly accounts for some, although not all, changes in functional, physical, and mental health.

Outcomes from a preliminary uncontrolled study with 24 breast-cancer survivors participating in eight-session PSIT groups[26] showed significant improvement in physical, emotional, and functional well-being scales as well as a meaning/peace subscale of spiritual well-being. Participants improved on mental-health measures of mood, including total mood disturbance and vigor, with significant decreases in depression, anger, fatigue, and tension. Participants improved on measures of posttraumatic growth, especially in apprehending new possibilities and personal strength, which illustrates the paradoxical benefit of empowerment gained from collaborative spiritual surrender. These preliminary studies suggest that PSIT may improve physical, functional, mental, and spiritual well-being and stimulate posttraumatic growth in cancer survivors.

To establish a clearer picture of the health and well-being effects of PSIT, it would be beneficial to conduct larger controlled studies. PSIT includes multiple spiritual practices that show substantial evidence of enhancing health and well-being. These include mindful meditation,[27] hatha yoga (see Park, Lee, Finkelstein-Fox, and Sanderson in this book), mantra meditation (see Pelletier and Bormann in this book), and self-compassion practices.[28] (For further descriptions of PSIT, see Wall, Corwin, and Koopman[29]; Corwin, Wall, and Koopman[30]; Wall, Nye, and FitzMedrud[31]; and Wall, Warner, FitzMedrud, and Meritt.[28])

PSIT emphasizes a personal experience of the sacred; therefore, it is suitable for people of most spiritual/religious traditions or none. This approach in PSIT elicited profound spiritual surrender experiences in Velasco-Scott's research[9] with an ethnically and religiously diverse sample: two Buddhists, five Catholics, one kriya yogi, one Unitarian, and four with no religious affiliation. Ethnically, this same sample consisted of one Chinese, one Eurasian, two Latinas, one Filipina, and seven Caucasians. This sample was selected for clear articulation of their surrender experience on open-ended questionnaires collected immediately after two separate guided surrender practices during PSIT sessions. Participants were asked to describe their immediate and previous experiences of surrender. The next section presents the process of PSIT for these cancer survivors and the personal descriptions of several surrender experiences as recorded in Velasco-Scott's qualitative research,[9] illustrating multiple qualities of spiritual surrender.

Psycho-Spiritual Integrative Therapy Processes, Including Spiritual Surrender

Psycho-Spiritual Integrative Therapy incorporates several spiritual practices culminating in spiritual surrender. In this section, we describe PSIT as it was conducted during an eight-week group therapy for cancer survivors.

PSIT begins with an exploration of the clients' highest spiritual aspirational purpose for their lives, which is a quality of spiritual surrender. Clients use meditation to develop nonjudgmental self-acceptance, labeled "witness." They then explore a personal sense of the sacred by sharing a passage from scripture or poetry that represents a personal comprehension of the Divine and then use a phrase from it as a mantra or prayer. Participants practice meditation with this personal mantra/prayer and are guided through a process that encourages them to experience spiritual surrender. This process includes physical movement from one standing position to another in order to shift conscious attention and "step" into a spiritually surrendered state. Participants depict their experiences in journals immediately after each experience and share their experiences with group members and the facilitator. Spiritual surrender allows participants to explore how they can take "next steps" to dedicate their lives to live more consistently in alignment with their higher life purposes. These planned "next steps" are shared with group members and the facilitator in order to publicly commit to their actualization.

Some clients report difficulties with spiritual surrender, as described by PSIT participants below. It is helpful to address difficulties in several ways. First, help clients to develop a broader collaborative definition of surrender and to experience a sense of enlargement from support of the Divine rather than one of defeat or giving. For this purpose, passages and/or poems from multiple spiritual traditions depicting the collaborative approach to spiritual surrender are read and discussed in PSIT. The exploration of spiritual surrender is not rushed or forced, as clients are encouraged to view surrender as a developmental process. Counselors facilitate present-moment awareness, mindfulness, self-acceptance, self-compassion, calmness, and peacefulness based on a common human experience of oneness. Counselors realize that people may experience the Divine as immanent, indwelling Divine; transcendent in the form of a beloved higher power, God/Jesus/Prophet; as universal, such as the prime mover or the power of nature; or they may have experiences of all three in spiritual surrender.

These PSIT processes are repeated in sessions and at home several times over the eight-week intervention. Surrender comes after a process of bringing awareness to a personalized sense of the sacred, thus allowing an evolving appraisal of the role of spirituality and spiritual life purpose in the participants' lives. These processes can encourage reappraisal and transcendent meaning making in recovery from cancer, since in PSIT spiritual surrender focuses on a person's multidimensional lived transcendent experience, not just beliefs or cognitive interpretations.

Below we present accounts of surrender experiences of cancer survivors participating in PSIT research groups[9] to explicate the nuanced qualities of surrender. Pseudonyms are used to protect confidentiality.

Sonya: Fear to Freedom, Regaining a Spiritual Connection

In PSIT, spiritual surrender is described as a collaborative alignment of one's personal will with Divine will, and as demonstrated below, it resulted for Sonya in a paradoxical sense of empowerment in coping with her cancer where she began to reap the fruits of surrender through an enlivened, purposeful life.

Sonya, a breast- cancer survivor in her fifties, declared no active religious/spiritual affiliation upon entry to the PSIT group. She had difficulty with spiritual surrender, which she described as a struggle. She stated that her emotions in the process were fear and anxiety. However, she had the insight to acknowledge that surrender was a process that could benefit her: "This concept of surrender is bringing up issues of trust and seems to open up a 'little girl' place of fear and sadness."

Initially she pushed herself to feel the willingness to surrender but fought it: "The very fiber of my body vibrates and resonates resistance to trust/surrender." She was highly frustrated with the concept and process of surrender: "I lose concentration. I want to run away and hide from surrender. It is taking powerful will to sit and write. I want to leave." Subsequently, she wrote in a second administration of an open-ended questionnaire that there was value in the process that she hoped would come to her in time: "I am making progress; fear is present to the word surrender. Curiosity and calling forth mature understanding that I am safe, helps."

Her struggles with conceptualizing to what or whom she surrendered stemmed from her inability to sense a higher power at first. To her, a higher power did not exist, and she could not let go of that. As a young adult, she did have a sense of belief in a higher power and experience of spirituality, but she was currently no longer connected:

> Yes, I believed in a higher power, a spirit, and ancestral spirit. That's gone, and I no longer feel connected. The organic elements have replaced the spiritual elements. I'm disappointed and feel cut free. Freedom is lonely. I can only now begin to sense a connection, [to my spiritual world] but I can't quite catch it. I want to have a spiritual grounding, but it is so very elusive and fragile. Surrender before [PSIT] group was completely out of reach! . . . not even within my vocabulary . . . an insensible concept. Now I see it something less questionable, and as a place where I can go to for rest. Trust, surrender, collapsed distinctions.

In her follow-up interview, Sonya explained that several traumatic events had happened several years prior to her cancer diagnosis, including the deaths of loved ones and career difficulties. These led to an inability to trust in benevolent spiritual support. Yet Sonya had some resolution of her conflicts and struggled with her scientific training, which had distanced her from spirituality. Sonya stated that she was able to learn deeper coping skills in PSIT, including spiritual surrender, which helped her move to a deeper place of peace and surrender:

> Yeah it is, it is very exciting! And, I recognize that it's a choice . . . that this stark reality that I've been living in, this black-and-white scientific world was one choice, but there was another choice, and the other choice is softer and a lot more pleasurable . . . so I lived in this stark, rough, overexposed, seared type of reality, or I can go into the . . . much more relaxed, easier deep breathing . . . visionary, create my own way, and that's what I've chosen. And I was able to access this through [PSIT] group.

At the beginning of the PSIT process, Sonya felt disconnected from her childhood spiritual connection, but she gradually gained a fragile essence of spirituality as she struggled with the idea and practice of spiritual surrender. As the process continued, she overcame barriers and reincorporated her connection to a personal sense of spirituality and was ultimately able to surrender. This resulted in a movement from what she described as a "seared type of reality" to a sense of agency in formulating a life of ease and creativity.

Debbie: From Pleading to Collaborative Spiritual Surrender

In this account, we see movement from pleading to collaborative surrender. Debbie's experience before the PSIT group was one in which she was pleading/praying for a personally defined outcome. Debbie, a Eurasian, had been a cancer survivor for seven months upon entry into the PSIT group. She had a Catholic background and had changed to Unity. She was in her mid-forties when she was diagnosed with stage II breast cancer. This diagnosis before age 50 is indicative of a poorer prognosis, adding to her distress. Debbie reported what she sincerely thought was surrender when she received her diagnosis, yet she used a pleading coping style that masqueraded as surrender. Debbie articulated the use of her will and pleading for a personal, desired outcome. Her thoughts and feelings were that surrender was to hope that she would "become well enough to tell her story of recuperation from cancer." Debbie was also relying on her personal willpower to purge the negative:

> I surrendered my condition as being unstable, *but the force of my will was stronger to overcome any obstacle.* I surrendered truly to God and his blessing. Every day I became closer to a universal presence and leaned on it for support, allowing the light of healing rays to touch every component of my being. *I purged negativity* out of *my mind, body, and soul and wished to become*

lighter, less dense so that the illness could dissipate into the ethers. [emphasis added]

After repeated practices of collaborative spiritual surrender in the PSIT sessions and home practice, Debbie found surrender infused with love and Christ consciousness. Debbie stated that she surrendered to

> love at a deeper level. The polarities . . . melt into one . . . making myself feel light and unbelievably solid at the same time. It is an acceptance of the universal and earthly love. The two spheres of the ephemeral and three-dimensional realities merge "on earth as it is in heaven." My Christ consciousness is elevated, and an all-encompassing cocoon of light and wisdom is now at a constant stream.

Debbie reported that instead of struggling with her physical condition of instability, she was able to accept it. She stated that her surrender experience caused her to move into an attitude in which "things seemed to flow better and nonjudgmental of myself [sic] and others." This self-acceptance supported her in her surrender of everything. She appeared to feel empowered by the act of collaborative surrender and find transcendent meaning in her life, whether her life situation appeared positive or negative. This illustrates transcendent "meanings-made" as a sense of a life of spiritually directed purpose, which is a quality of a collaborative spiritual surrender. In Debbie's situation, we see healthy movement from pleading to a collaborative spiritual surrender and transformative immersion in Christ consciousness, which is in a "constant stream," perhaps reflecting dedication to a spiritual life purpose. Debbie demonstrated the ability to reappraise the meaning of surrender and adapted to the more health-promoting collaborative approach.

These intimate accounts vividly illustrate qualities of spiritual surrender and the exponential shifts in motivations, values, perceptions, and realizations of a greater life purpose. Some cancer survivors credited PSIT processes for providing methods to overcome barriers and gain spiritual tools in order to cope. Many felt they would reap the benefits throughout their lives. We are grateful to the PSIT participants who shared their personal transformative experiences and hope PSIT and the practice of spiritual surrender have long-lasting impacts on their well-being.

Conclusion

Many spiritual traditions recommend spiritual surrender as a means of relieving suffering and living a spiritually purposeful, healthy life. Collaborative spiritual surrender aligns the personal and the Divine will: do what you can and accept God's support for the uncontrollable. The evidence of spiritual surrender's positive effects on health and well-being for people suffering with physical illness is promising yet sparse. Only a few small studies of spiritually integrated psychotherapies incorporating collaborative spiritual surrender as one of several spiritual practices have demonstrated positive results. Though these results are promising, they are preliminary. Larger, randomized trials would enhance our understanding of the health effects of surrender in counseling.

Important qualities of spiritual surrender are found in larger quantitative research on religious/spiritual coping styles and spiritual meaning making when people are seriously ill. Coping research indicates that collaborative spiritual surrender increases well-being in comparison to a religious/spiritual practice of pleading for a personally defined outcome or deferring all responsibility to the Divine. Collaborative spiritual surrender is especially potent for people in situations of high stress where personal control is restrained, such as those suffering from serious illnesses. Patients who resolve struggles and make meaning of the existential and spiritual issues arising from their illness are more likely to have positive adjustments and growth than those who continue the search for meaning.

Seriously ill people who persist in using negative religious/spiritual practices and beliefs (e.g., deferring coping rather than collaborative spiritual surrender) may have accelerated disability in comparison to those who either initially exhibit or change to positive spiritual practices such as collaborative spiritual surrender. Fortunately, people are capable of adopting positive spiritual beliefs and collaborative spiritual surrender as exemplified in the rich personal accounts of cancer survivors participating in Psycho-Spiritual Integrative Therapy presented in this chapter. Repeated practice of collaborative spiritual surrender yields many positive gifts of serenity, spiritual life purpose, motivation to increase health, and spiritual well-being. We hope this chapter will encourage additional studies and counseling applications inclusive of spiritual surrender to assist people in realizing the health benefits and transformative aspects of this profound spiritual practice.

References

1. O'Brian, Y. E. G. (2016). *Living for the sake of the soul*. San Jose, CA: CSE Press.

2. Cole, B., & Pargament, K. (1999). Spiritual surrender: A paradoxical path to control. In W. Miller (Ed.), *Integrating spirituality into treatment: Resources for practitioners* (pp. 179–188). Washington, DC: American Psychological Association.

3. Koenig, H. G., Pargament, K. I., & Nielsen, J. (1998). Religious coping and health status in medically ill, hospitalized older adults. *Journal of Nervous and Mental Diseases, 186,* 513–521.

4. Pargament, K., Kennell, J., Hathaway, W., Grevengoed, N., Newman, J., & Jones, W. (1988). Religion and the problem solving process: Three styles of coping. *Journal for the Scientific Study of Religion, 27,* 90–104.

5. Pargament, K., Ensing, D., Falgout, K., Olsen, H., Reilly, G., Van Haitsma, K., & Warren, R. (1990). God help me (I): Religious coping efforts as predictors of the outcomes of significant negative life events. *American Journal of Community Psychology, 18,* 793–824.

6. Pargament, K. (1997). *The psychology of religion and coping: Theory, research, practice.* New York: Guilford Press.

7. Gunnlaugson, O., & Moze, M. B. (2012). Surrendering into witnessing: A foundational practice for building collective intelligence capacity in groups. *Journal of Integral Theory and Practice, 7*(30), 105–115.

8. Aurobindo, Sri. (2000/1958). *Letters on yoga* (Vols. 1–5). Pondicherry, India: Sri Aurobindo Ashram. (Original work published 1958.)

9. Velasco-Scott, S. (2015). The experience of spiritual surrender in cancer survivors participating in Psycho-Spiritual Integrative Therapy (PSIT). ProQuest Dissertations Publishing, 3709231.

10. Clements, A. D., & Ermakova, A. V. (2012). Surrender to God and stress: A possible link between religiosity and health. *Psychology of Religion and Spirituality, 4,* 93–107. http://dx.doi.org/doi:10.1037/a0025109

11. Wong-McDonald, A., & Gorsuch, R. (2000). Surrender to God: An additional coping style? *Journal of Psychology and Theology, 28,* 149–161.

12. Pargament, K., Koenig, H., Tarakeshwar, N., & Hahn, J. (2004). Religious coping methods as predictors of psychological, physical and spiritual outcomes among medically ill elderly patients: A two-year longitudinal study. *Journal of Health Psychology, 6,* 713–730.

13. Park, C. (2013). The meaning making model: A framework for understanding meaning, spirituality, and stress-related growth in health psychology. *European Health Psychologist, 15*(2), 40–47.

14. Yanez, B., Edmondson, D., Stanton, A. L., Park, C. L., Kwan, L., Ganz, P. A., & Blank, T. O. (2009). Facets of spirituality as predictors of adjustment to cancer: Relative contributions of having faith and finding meaning. *Journal of Consulting and Clinical Psychology, 77*(4), 730–741.

15. Jim, H. S., & Andersen, B. L. (2007). Meaning in life mediates the relationship between social and physical functioning and distress in cancer survivors. *British Journal of Health Psychology, 12,* 363–381.

16. Segerstrom, S. C., Stanton, A. L., Alden, L. E., & Shortridge, B. E. (2003). A multidimensional structure for repetitive thought: What's on your mind, and how, and how much? *Journal of Personality and Social Psychology, 85,* 909–921. doi:10.1037/0022-3514.85.5.909

17. Cole, B. S., Hopkins, C. M., Tisak, J., Steel, J. L., & Carr, B. I. (2008). Assessing spiritual growth and spiritual decline following a diagnosis of cancer: Reliability and validity of the spiritual transformation scale. *Psycho-Oncology, 17,* 112–121. doi:10.1002/pon.1207

18. Park, C. L., Edmondson, D., Hale-Smith, A., & Blank, T. O. (2009). Religiousness/spirituality and health behaviors in younger adult cancer survivors: Does faith promote healthier lifestyles? *Journal of Behavioral Medicine, 32,* 582–591. doi:10:1007/s10865-009-9223-6

19. Pargament, K., Kennell, J., Hathaway, W., Grevengoed, N., Newman, J., & Jones, W. (1988). Religion and the problem solving process: Three styles of coping. *Journal for the Scientific Study of Religion, 27,* 90–104.

20. Tarakeshwar, N., Pearce, M. J., & Sikkema, K. J. (2005). Development and implementation of a spiritual coping group intervention for adults living with HIV/AIDS: A pilot study. *Mental Health, Religion and Culture, 8*(3), 179–190. http://dx.doi.org/10.1080/13694670500138908

21. Cole, B. S., & Pargament, K. I. (1999). Re-Creating Your Life: A spiritual /psychotherapy for people diagnosed with cancer. *Psychooncology, 8*(5), 395–407.

22. Cole, B. S. (2005). Spiritually-focused psychotherapy for people diagnosed with cancer: A pilot outcome study. *Mental Health, Religion and Culture, 8*(3), 217–226.

23. Cole, B., Pargament, K. I., & Brownstein, S. (2000). A cognitive-behavioral group intervention for cardiac syncope. Paper presented at the Annual Meeting of the American Psychological Association, Washington, D.C. In K. I. Pargament. (2002). God help me: Advances in the psychology of religion and coping. *Archives for the Psychology of Religion, 24,* 48–63.

24. Rosequist, L., Wall, K., Corwin, D., Achterberg, J., & Koopman, C. (2012). Surrender as a form of active acceptance among breast cancer survivors receiving Psycho-Spiritual Integrative Therapy. *Support Care Cancer, 20,* 2821–2827. doi:10.1007/s00520-012-1406-y

25. Johnson, A. V. (2011). An investigation of spiritual mediators of quality of life and mood among cancer survivors participating in Psycho-Spiritual Integrative Therapy. *Dissertation Abstracts International: Section B. Sciences and Engineering, 73*(6), 0669.

26. Garlick, M., Wall, K., Corwin, D., & Koopman, C. (2011). Psycho-Spiritual Integrative Therapy for women with primary breast cancer. *Journal of Clinical Psychology in Medical Settings, 1,* 78–90. http://dx.doi.org/doi:10.1007/s10880-011-9224-9

27. Gotink, R. A., Chu, P., Busschbach, J. J. V., Benson, H., Fricchione, G. L., & Hunink, M. G. M. (2015). Standardized mindfulness-based interventions in healthcare: An overview of systematic reviews and meta-analyses of RCTs. *PLoS ONE, 10*(4), e0124344. doi:10.1371/journal.pone.0124344

28. Wall, K., Warner, A., FitzMedrud, E., & Meritt, K. (2015). Self-compassion in psychotherapy: A Psycho-Spiritual Integrative Therapy approach. In T. G. Plante (Ed.), *The psychology of compassion and cruelty: Understanding the emotional, spiritual, and religious influences* (pp. 173–190). Santa Barbara, CA: Praeger.

29. Wall, K., Corwin, C., & Koopman, C. (2012). Reaping fruits of spirituality through Psycho-Spiritual Integrative Therapy in cancer recovery. In T. G. Plante (Ed.), *Religion and positive psychology: Understanding the psychological fruits of faith* (pp. 233–246). Santa Barbara, CA: Praeger.

30. Corwin, D., Wall, K., & Koopman, C. (2012). Psycho-Spiritual Integrative Therapy: Psychological intervention for women with breast cancer. *The Journal for Specialists in Group Work, 37*(3), 252–273. doi:10.1080/01933922.2012.686961

31. Wall, K., Nye, F., & FitzMedrud, E. (2013). Psychospiritual integrative practices. In H. Friedman & G. Hartelius (Eds.), *The Wiley-Blackwell handbook of transpersonal psychology* (pp. 544–561). Chichester, UK: Wiley-Blackwell. doi:10.1002/9781118591277

Yoga to Promote Physical, Mental, and Spiritual Well-Being: Self-Regulation on and off the Mat

Crystal L. Park, Sharon Y. Lee,
Lucy Finkelstein-Fox,
and Kalliope Sanderson

As typically practiced in the West, yoga is a mind-body practice involving postures, breath work, and meditation. Yoga's increasing popularity has been matched by an increasing body of scientific literature assessing its effectiveness in promoting physical and mental health and well-being. In this chapter, we provide background on how yoga has developed in the West and review how yoga promotes physical, mental, and spiritual well-being through enhancing self-regulation (i.e., improving emotional, cognitive, and behavioral regulation). Because yoga promotes self-regulation, which is essential for mental and physical health, it is a beneficial practice for improving well-being that can be used as a stand-alone intervention or an adjunct to other therapies. We provide suggestions for translating yoga teachings to daily life and specific recommendations for health-care providers.

Evolution of Yoga

Yoga Is Increasing in Prevalence and Visibility

Originating in India, yoga is an ancient set of practices designed to promote spiritual, emotional, physical, and psychological well-being. Yoga practice typically encompasses multiple components, including physical movement, breath work, sensory withdrawal or meditation, and ethical discipline. As practiced in the Western hemisphere, yoga is often most heavily based on its physical components (*asana*) but also includes some components of breathing, meditation, or mindfulness. As of this writing, rates of yoga practice in the United States have reached an all-time high; a 2016 estimate was that nearly 37 million Americans have practiced yoga at least once, which represents a large increase from the 20.4 million who reported practicing four years earlier in 2012.[1] Further, these rates may be even higher among specific groups, such as those with health issues[2] or those who identify with certain religions, such as Buddhism.[3]

More and more, it seems that yoga is *everywhere*. Many gyms and specialized studios hold frequent yoga classes, billed as a form of wellness promotion, stretching, or relaxation. Yoga that focuses on physical strength and cardiovascular endurance, such as ashtanga, vinyasa, power yoga, and Bikram, is especially popular in these settings. Many holistic wellness centers and counseling services also offer yoga, often framed as a stress-management practice that incorporates aspects of meditation, mindfulness, relaxation, and/or gentle stretching. Outside of these group classes, many individuals practice yoga on their own, making use of popular YouTube channels, mobile apps, or other online streaming services provided for free or for a cost. Indeed, the high demand for yoga in the West, coupled with a huge spike in mobile technology, has resulted in a vast business of yoga within the larger "wellness" culture. Because yoga practice is by nature highly individualized and modifiable, it holds great potential for improving health and well-being.

Yoga as Spiritual Practice

As originally practiced in India, yoga comprises eight limbs: *asana* (physicality), *yama* (ethical practice), *niyama* (individual observances), *pranayama* (breath), *pratyahara* (withdrawal of senses), *dharana* (concentration), *dhyana* (mindfulness/meditation), and *samadhi* (self-realization/enlightenment). Clearly, although Western yoga practice often emphasizes physicality, spiritual and ethical rituals are also an essential element of traditional yoga. A central theme of these individual components is the separation from external distraction and emphasis on meaningful engagement with oneself and one's community, ultimately moving toward a state of enlightenment.

Of note, the spiritual aspects of yoga appear to exist independent of any one established religion. Although yoga is an important element of religions commonly practiced in India, such as Hinduism, Buddhism, and Jainism, individuals from other religious or spiritual belief systems (e.g., Christianity) as well as individuals who identify as nonreligious may also use yoga practice as a ritualistic means of achieving greater spiritual well-being.[4]

Although research linking yoga practice to changes in spirituality is lacking, some studies have suggested that mindfulness, an important aspect of many yoga practices, may be linked to increases in spiritual well-being, especially with regard to having a sense of meaning and peace rather than religious faith.[5] Thus, mindfulness may represent a mechanism through which yoga enhances personal spirituality, regardless of one's specific religious identity; the universal and multidimensional nature of mindfulness is discussed further by Shapiro and von Garnier in chapter 3, this volume.

Yoga as Exercise

In the West, yoga has increasingly been incorporated into mainstream "wellness" culture since the 1990s. Many people first experience yoga in a group fitness class setting where the primary focus is on physical *asana* and breathing rather than on spirituality. Even for those with limited access to a gym or yoga studio membership, an *asana*-focused home practice is highly accessible via online resources, mobile applications, or solo practice.

Although many yoga classes include a brief meditation or mindfulness exercise at the beginning, and/or a brief meditative *savasana* (relaxation/corpse pose) at the close of practice, physicality is often the hallmark of practice. Serving as exercise, yoga produces direct health benefits, including increased flexibility, strength building, and cardiovascular fitness. Further, as with other forms of exercise, benefits may come through indirect pathways, such as stress reduction, self-compassion, and improvements in eating and exercise behaviors and sleep. Some yoga teachers have even added nontraditional elements to their classes to increase students' caloric expenditure; these might include heated rooms, small weights, or standard core strengthening (e.g., crunches).

In addition to the strength-building and cardiovascular benefits associated with yoga practice, the use of yoga classes for stretching and recovery from physical injury or soreness among athletes has received attention. Endorsement by professional athletes of the benefits of stretching has added to the conceptualization of yoga as an important aspect of physical fitness. The importance of building flexibility and strength is similarly emphasized in older adults (discussed by Richards and DiMartino in chapter 7, this volume) as well as other populations with physical limitations.

Yoga as Treatment

Because yoga is so often associated with increased wellness, it is not surprising that both behavioral health and primary care clinicians have attempted to capitalize on its accessibility and acceptability in suggesting yoga practice to their patients. Randomized controlled trials have provided preliminary evidence that yoga practice may lead to small to moderate reductions in symptoms of chronic pain, including low back pain,[6] fibromyalgia, and arthritis;[7] however, more high-quality research studies on these effects are sorely needed. Yoga has also begun to demonstrate efficacy in managing high blood pressure and other cardiovascular disease risk factors, characterized by improvements in lung capacity, oxygen delivery, VO_2 and respiration rate, and resting heart rate.[8] Further, a small number of studies have suggested that yoga may improve symptoms of irritable bowel syndrome, another stress-related condition, although further research is needed to support these findings.[9] As noted above, yoga also represents a promising method of promoting weight-loss efforts among individuals who are overweight or obese.[10] Despite the significant limitations of the existing research, however, yoga appears to be highly acceptable to many people and may be a promising complementary modality for improving physical symptoms.

Yoga has also demonstrated preliminary efficacy in reducing stress, anxiety, and depression, as demonstrated by improvements in immune functioning, GABA, and salivary cortisol as well as self-reported symptoms.[11] Studies have demonstrated that yoga may be a promising adjunctive treatment for posttraumatic stress disorder, with small to medium effect sizes on clinician-administered tests and self-reported symptoms.[12] Yoga may also be an important method of stress reduction for individuals with one or more serious chronic medical conditions (see chapter 7, this volume, for a discussion of yoga for multiple chronic conditions) and has demonstrated moderate to large effects on psychological well-being and general quality of life in research with cancer patients, with smaller effects on physical functioning (see chapter 14, this volume, for a description of moving meditation interventions for cancer patients).[13] Importantly, although it appears that yoga may lead to significant improvements when compared to placebo or no treatment, the existing evidence for its effects on psychological symptoms is insufficient to make comparisons to other evidence-based treatments. Still, yoga is increasingly being used as an adjunct treatment for people undergoing cancer treatments and people in recovery programs for substance abuse and has demonstrated a high degree of acceptability among patients and providers.

A Self-Regulation Perspective on Yoga

Many of the beneficial effects of yoga on physical, mental, and spiritual well-being can be attributed to its fostering of greater capacity for self-regulation. Self-regulation refers to "the way that a person controls his or her own responses so as to pursue or maintain goals and live up to standards" (p. 500).[14] In other words, self-regulation refers to one's capacity to override an incipient response and thereby permit a preferred alternative. Self-regulation involves four main elements: standards, monitoring, motivation, and willpower.[15] In sum, self-regulation involves having a chosen set of guidelines, an ability to observe one's behaviors relative to those guidelines, and the desire and ability to override responses that are ultimately less desirable.

Self-regulation is a continuous process of attempting to use information about one's current state to monitor and, when necessary, change that state in order to move toward one's goals. Self-regulation can occur in the domains of cognition, emotion, and behavior (see Figure 6.1). Cognitive self-regulation is directed at executive functions such as goal representation, attentional stability and control, concentration, thought suppression or reappraisal, focus of awareness, self-monitoring, and working memory. Emotional self-regulation refers to the management of the experience of emotions and inner states and can involve increasing, decreasing, or maintaining particular emotions, both positive and negative. Behavioral self-regulation involves guiding or adjusting one's behavior in pursuit of desired end states or goals. Behavioral self-regulation encompasses a range of behaviors, such as resisting temptation, overriding impulses, employing and overriding habits, selecting or avoiding

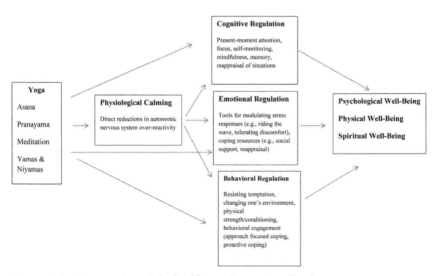

Figure 6.1   Proposed Model of Self-Regulatory Benefits from Yoga

particular situations, and responding to situational demands with various types of approach-focused (actively dealing with one's stressors) and proactive coping (taking actions to avoid stressors before they happen).[16]

Self-regulation of cognitions, emotions, and behaviors is vitally important for overall psychological, physical, and spiritual well-being, including building and maintaining interpersonal relationships, regulating impulses, keeping stress levels low, making decisions that are consistent with one's belief systems, and engaging in healthy lifestyles: essentially, for living the life one wants to live. However, individuals vary widely in their ability to self-regulate, with many individuals having substantial deficits in their regulatory abilities.[17] Failures in self-regulation can lead to aggression, violence, substance abuse, depression, and anxiety disorders, and the resultant stress and poor health behaviors can lead to a host of physical health problems.[17]

Many aspects of yoga practice help to develop and support self-regulation,[18] including meditative movement, conscious breathing, body and emotion awareness, open curiosity, attention allocation, self-compassion, and acceptance.[16] Through these aspects of yoga, practitioners can strengthen their capacity for emotional stability and equanimity, an even-minded mental state or dispositional tendency toward all experience regardless of its affective valence or source. Through continued practice, yoga can help individuals cultivate more adaptive and fewer maladaptive cognitions, emotions, and behaviors. In combination, these different aspects of yoga make it a highly potent intervention for improving self-regulation capacity. The more that practitioners practice yoga, the greater their tendency for adaptive self-regulation, both on and off the yoga mat.

Yoga conceptualizes the self as multidimensional and offers several pathways with associated techniques from which to tailor a personal practice. Yoga is thus very adaptable to meet the needs of individual students where they are psychologically as well physically. This particular quality also makes yoga approachable across time and culture. In addition, while yogic techniques are practiced synergistically "on the mat," many of them can be applied "off the mat" (see Table 6.1). Thus, yoga supports experimenting with self-regulation in the laboratory of practice and also in the midst of living.

Yoga's Tools for Self-Regulation: Postures, Breath, and Meditation

Although each of the eight limbs of yoga provides tools that increase self-regulation, we focus here specifically on five of the eight limbs that collectively form the three basic elements of yoga—postures, breathing techniques, and the three meditative limbs (sensory withdrawal, concentration, and meditative absorption). As noted above, these five limbs make up most Western yoga classes. Effects of the five limbs discussed below are further outlined in our proposed model of yoga for self-regulation (Figure 6.1).

Table 6.1   Yoga and Self-Regulation on and off the Mat

Practical Strategy	Application
Awareness, concentration, steady mind	• Set an intention • Find your growing edge • Still eyes help still the mind • Return focus again and again • Keep your eyes on your own mat
Tolerating and accepting discomfort	• Stay when you feel like leaving • Learn to be comfortable with the discomfort • Everything is temporary and all will pass • It is already okay
Non-judgment	• Find the inner witness: self-objectivity (fire the judge, hire the witness) • Approach feelings of stress with curiosity, non- judgment (just notice) • Watch thoughts come and go (like watching traffic go by) without engaging them
Centering	• Stitch half-breaths together • You carry your breath with you (you are your own "regulator") • Slowing down breath slows down nervous system • Find a centering point during moments of rapid thoughts • Still your eyes, still your mind (drishti)

Postures (Asana)

Traditionally, postures, or *asanas*, are practiced to increase life-force energy, or *prana*. The yoga practitioner moves the body through different postures to release physical and mental tension, bring various biological systems into balance, and enhance flexibility,[19] which, in turn, enables the mind to become steady and focused.

Breathing Techniques (Pranayama)

The Upanishads, an ancient yogic text, describes *prana* as "the principle of life and consciousness." *Pranayama*, translated as "prolongation of breath and its restraint" is an essential part of yoga practice and of self-regulation.[20]

Pranayama practices are thought to help bring the mind and the body into balance and are practiced either on their own or in combination with postures. Practicing various breathing exercises can teach practitioners about the relationship between how they breathe and how they feel. In particular, cultivating *ujjayi* breath—long, slow inhales and exhales—is soothing to the central nervous system. In many yoga classes, students are invited to practice this slow, deep breath as they also practice and move through the postures. Thus, *pranayama* can become a valuable tool for calming oneself in stressful situations.

Meditation

The various forms of meditation promoted by yoga are key tools in the regulation of the mind. For example, Kripalu yoga emphasizes witness consciousness, the ability to observe experience without reaction. Witness consciousness can be likened to the more recently popularized concept of mindfulness. In yoga class, students will be guided into a pose and invited to deepen their breath and then to witness (be mindful of) their experience.

In the course of everyday life, yoga practitioners will encounter challenges and stressors that call for a response, and it is in this context that many of the skills acquired in yoga practice can be used for self-regulation. Our model posits that yoga practice can improve cognitive, emotional, and behavioral aspects of self-regulation. Many yoga practices can facilitate better cognitive regulation. As noted above, meditation is a central aspect of yoga; in fact, yoga is often called "meditation in motion." Regular practice allows individuals to learn to focus their thinking on a single point. Attention in *asana* is often directed to a specific part of one's body (e.g., ball of foot, fingertips); similarly, *pranayama* involves focusing on the breath as it moves through the body. In essence, the body is a central object of meditation within many yoga practices. Therefore, interoceptive feedback from the very object of meditation may be an important, and distinctive, feature of yoga relative to other forms of meditation. These experiences give students practical experience in objects of meditation, and the resultant attention skills can promote cognitive regulation by helping individuals avoid ruminative thoughts and focus their attention on other, less stressful objects.

This embodiment suggests that mindful yoga, or a practice in which students are encouraged to attend closely to their present experience without judgment, may offer additional tools for some populations that sitting meditation alone cannot provide. For example, mindful yoga may be more suited to those with chronic illness than is meditation alone. Yoga may support chronic illness schema change by challenging beliefs about the limits of one's physical body. As students practice poses and stretch the body in ways they might not have felt they could, they may come to see that while some aspects of their bodies are limited, other parts of the body are still healthy.

Yoga practice can improve emotion regulation through several pathways, as outlined in Figure 6.1. One of these is mindfulness; witnessing one's experience, rather than trying to modify it or psychologically understand it, is believed to help practitioners break through distressing thoughts and emotions. Yoga offers a forum in which to practice mindfulness again and again. Positive reappraisal is another important emotion-regulation skill that can be enhanced by yoga: much of yoga practice involves learning to reframe experiences (e.g., from labeling an experience *discomfort* to labeling it *sensation*), teaching a more objective, observational, and nonjudgmental stance to one's experience. Other reappraisal resources can be acquired through yoga practice. For example, in the course of yoga classes, teachers often instruct students about deeper aspects of yoga philosophy, such as compassion and impermanence, which are useful in appraising or reappraising situations as less stressful. Many types of yoga promote being present for one's emotional experiences.

Yoga may improve behavioral self-regulation by increasing self-awareness, a critical component of self-regulation,[15] allowing individuals to clearly compare their current status vis-à-vis their goals and to make any necessary behavioral adjustments. Yoga practice teaches more deliberate and mindful actions, giving individuals practice in overcoming impulsive temptations. Yoga practice may also help individuals to limit their stress exposure by being aware of their limits and employing proactive coping strategies to prevent exposure to excessive stress.

How Does Yoga Promote Self-Regulation?

Yoga provides a context in which people can learn and practice self-regulation skills, which they can then take "off the mat" and into the rest of their lives. The *yamas* and *niyamas* referred to above comprise 10 ethical guidelines or standards of behavior. Rather than being considered rules or laws, they can be viewed as invitations to act in ways that promote inner and outer peace and happiness. The first *yama*, for example, is *ahimsa* (nonviolence). Some of these principles can be practiced on the mat, but many are meant to be enacted primarily outside of yoga class. For example, *brahmacharya* advocates practicing moderation and self-restraint.

The monitoring function of yoga can be seen in the self-inquiry that yoga encourages. Much of yoga practice involves observing oneself in a nonattached, nonjudgmental way, finding one's deep inner witness and watching the external self-interact with the environment. Motivation for monitoring and adaptively changing behavior comes from an enhanced desire for higher self-actualization that arises through continued and consistent practice.

Finally, the willpower to persist when making or maintaining changes is fostered by many aspects of yoga.

Yoga builds up willpower through consistent practice of overriding impulses and learning to simply breathe through difficult moments. For example, although some types of yoga are very gentle and soothing, many yoga traditions teach discipline and focus, encouraging individuals to get into and hold difficult poses that can create increasing discomfort as they are held longer. Rather than simply getting out of the pose when one wants to (assuming one's more superordinate goal is to stay in the pose), a goal of yoga is to look at the discomfort with a perspective of curiosity and non-judgment, to feel compassion for one's discomfort, and to continue to breathe and override the desire to leave the pose before the teacher gives the instruction to do so. Such practices provide yoga students with powerful and immediate demonstrations of their own self-regulatory abilities. In addition, yoga provides many resources that have been demonstrated in previous work to bolster self-regulatory abilities. For example, consistent practice can improve physical stamina and strength, self-confidence and self-efficacy, vitality and energy, sleep, and positive emotions as well as lower stress and negative affect, all of which have been shown to promote willpower.

Recommendations for Health-Care Providers

The self-regulatory benefits arising from yoga practice can be optimally leveraged when integrated into an individual's health maintenance and treatment plan. In addition to the direct benefits of self-regulatory skills arising from yoga practice, self-regulation is a significant predictor of many physical and mental health behaviors, including diet and medication adherence. In this way, self-regulatory skills developed through yoga practice can have both a direct and an indirect impact on physical, mental, and spiritual health and well-being. Health-care providers can play an integral role in maximizing these self-regulatory benefits for patients by making appropriate referrals and recommendations, encouraging patients to apply the principles of yoga to daily life, and encouraging continued yoga practice.

Promote the Practice of Yoga

Health-care providers can increase awareness of yoga and its benefits by making recommendations and referrals to patients. Many integrated care settings, such as Veterans Affairs medical centers and comprehensive cancer centers, have begun to offer yoga classes to their patients. Providers can also forge relationships with local yoga studios, particularly in settings where patients are seen in community-based clinics or practices. Research suggests that patients are likely to be receptive to such recommendations; there is mounting evidence that many patients who cope with physical or mental health issues are amenable to yoga.[21,22]

When making recommendations and referrals, providers should gauge the appropriateness of fit between the patient and style of yoga. Different styles of yoga may accommodate and address different mental and physical needs (see chapter 7, this volume, for examples of adapting yoga for older adults). The National Center for Complementary and Integrative Health acknowledges that, although side effects are rare, individuals with high blood pressure, glaucoma, and sciatica should take precautions by modifying or avoiding some poses.[23] Accordingly, providers can initiate conversations with patients about anticipating limitations (e.g., mobility), requesting accommodations (e.g., supportive props), and setting boundaries (e.g., no physical contact from teacher) in relation to patients' physical and mental health.

Apply Principles of Yoga Philosophy

Many of the principles of yoga philosophy are consistent with the principles that patients learn in psychotherapy. In fact, it could be argued that the *niyama* of *svadhyaya*, or self-study, aligns with the process of psychotherapy, from which patients develop insight into their maladaptive patterns of beliefs and behaviors. Therefore, mental health providers, such as psychologists, social workers, and pastoral counselors, are particularly well suited to facilitate discussions in which the principles learned in a patient's yoga practice are connected to concepts in psychotherapy. For example, psychotherapeutic approaches often talk about a patient's "inner critic," a personification of negative judgments about one's self. Patients can be reminded to manage their inner critics by applying the yogic principle of *ahimsa*, which espouses nonviolence and nonharm, to themselves.

In addition, one's yoga practice can be seen as a microcosm for one's way of relating to the world. As stated by one of B. K. S. Iyengar's disciples, Judith Hanson Lasater, "The whole world is your yoga mat."[24] Patients can process and extrapolate from their in-the-moment yoga experiences with mental health providers to develop strategies for managing stressful life situations. Patients can reflect on helpful strategies that were used while holding difficult poses (e.g., positive self-talk, reminders of the long-term benefits) and be encouraged to apply these strategies during stressful moments in daily life. The *niyama* of *tapas*, or self-discipline, aptly fits when patients are tolerating discomfort, pain, or distress during challenging situations, as is often the case for patients with physical or mental health conditions.

Encourage Use of Self-Regulatory Strategies

Providers can remind patients to practice self-regulatory strategies learned from yoga practice that provide immediate benefits for regulating physiological activity. Table 6.1 presents common concepts and phrases incorporated into yoga practice that can be translated off the mat and applied to self-regulatory efforts in everyday life. *Pranayama*, or controlled breathing exercises, can have short-term effects in regulating autonomic nervous system activity. Mindfulness and meditation are also components of yoga practice that have become increasing popular in psychotherapy applications, with evidence of lowering blood pressure and improving immune response.[25] Mental health providers can demonstrate and practice these strategies with patients in vivo by having patients rate how they feel before and after each exercise. Even for patients who do not practice yoga, the incorporation of basic yoga exercises such as *nadi shodhana pranayama*, or alternate-nostril breathing, may be a way of introducing the self-regulatory benefits of yoga to patients or clients who do not have ready access to regular yoga classes.

Reinforce the Benefits of Yoga

Inherent in the idea of yoga as a practice is the expectation that individuals will return to their mat regularly. Regular practice of yoga becomes self-regulatory behavior, as patients must organize their lives and regulate their behaviors in order to commit to their practice. Providers can reinforce regular yoga practice by praising patients for their commitment, providing feedback about observed benefits of yoga for the patient, and problem solving with patients when barriers interfere with regular practice. Yoga practice can also be reinforced using language consistent with psychotherapeutic concepts. Providers can frame yoga practice as part of a self-care routine for patients who are managing stress or behavioral activation for patients who are struggling with depression.

Conclusion

As yoga increases in popularity and accessibility, understanding the ways in which yoga's benefits translate from the mat to everyday life becomes more imperative. Many of the physical, mental, and spiritual benefits of yoga may be the function of improved self-regulatory abilities. Building these self-regulatory abilities may occur via emotional, cognitive, and behavioral processes. Considering the important role of self-regulation in determining health outcomes, health-care providers should consider recommending yoga as a way of increasing self-regulatory skills for patients.

References

1. Yoga Journal and Yoga Alliance. (2017, April 13). 2016 Yoga in America Study conducted by Yoga Journal and Yoga Alliance. Retrieved on October 23, 2017, from https://www.yogajournal.com/page/yogainamericastudy

2. Cramer, H., Ward, L., Steel, A., Lauche, R., Dobos, G., & Zhang, Y. (2016). Prevalence, patterns, and predictors of yoga use: Results of a US nationally representative survey. *American Journal of Preventive Medicine, 50,* 230–235.

3. Hasselle-Newcombe, S. (2005). Spirituality and "mystical religion" in contemporary society: A case of British practitioners of the Iyengar method of yoga. *Journal of Contemporary Religion, 20,* 305–322.

4. Büssing, A., Hedtstück, A., Khalsa, S. B. S., Ostermann, T., & Heusser, P. (2012). Development of specific aspects of spirituality during a 6-month intensive yoga practice. *Evidence-Based Complementary and Alternative Medicine, 2012,* Article ID: 981523. doi:10.1155/2012/981523

5. Carmody, J., Reed, G., Kristeller, J., & Merriam, P. (2008). Mindfulness, spirituality, and health-related symptoms. *Journal of Psychosomatic Research, 64,* 393–403.

6. Wieland, L.S., Skoetz, N., Pilkington, K., Vempati, R., D'Adamo, C.R., & Berman, B.M. (2017). Yoga treatment for chronic non-specific low back pain. *Cochrane Database of Systematic Reviews,* (1), Article ID: CD010671. doi:10.1002/14651858.CD010671.pub2

7. Ward, L., Stebbings, S., Cherkin, D., & Baxter, G. D. (2013). Yoga for functional ability, pain and psychosocial outcomes in musculoskeletal conditions: A systematic review and meta-analysis. *Musculoskeletal Care, 11,* 203–217.

8. Cramer, H., Haller, H., Lauche, R., Steckhan, N., Michalsen, A., & Dobos, G. (2014). A systematic review and meta-analysis of yoga for hypertension. *American Journal of Hypertension, 27*(9), 1146–1151.

9. Schumann, D., Anheyer, D., Lauche, R., Dobos, G., Langhorst, J., & Cramer, H. (2016). Effect of yoga in the therapy of irritable bowel syndrome: A systematic review. *Clinical Gastroenterology and Hepatology, 14,* 1720–1731.

10. Lauche, R., Langhorst, J., Lee, M. S., Dobos, G., & Cramer, H. (2016). A systematic review and meta-analysis on the effects of yoga on weight-related outcomes. *Preventative Medicine, 87,* 213–232.

11. Pascoe, M. C., & Bauer, I. E. (2015). A systematic review of randomized control trials on the effects of yoga on stress measures and mood. *Journal of Psychiatric Research, 68,* 270–282.

12. Gallegos, A. M., Crean, H. F., Pigeon, W. R., & Heffner, K. L. (2017). Meditation and yoga for posttraumatic stress disorder: A meta-analytic review of randomized controlled trials. *Clinical Psychology Review, 58,* 115–124.

13. Buffart, L. M., van Uffelen, J. G. Z., Riphagen, I. I., Burg, J., van Mechelen, W., Brown, W. J., & Chinapaw, M. J. M. (2012). Physical and psychosocial benefits of yoga in cancer patients and survivors, a systematic review and meta-analysis of randomized controlled trials. *BMC Cancer, 12,* 559.

14. Baumeister, R. F., & Vohs, K. D. (2007). Self-regulation, ego depletion, and motivation. *Social and Personality Psychology Compass, 1,* 115–128.

15. Zell, A. L., & Baumeister, R. F. (2013). How religion can support self-control and moral behavior. In R. F. Paloutzian & C. L. Park (Eds.), *Handbook of the psychology of religion and spirituality* (2nd ed.) (pp. 498–518). New York: Guilford Press.

16. Gard, T., Noggle, J. J., Park, C. L., Vago, D. R., & Wilson, A. (2014). Potential self-regulatory mechanisms of yoga for psychological health. *Frontiers in Human Neuroscience, 8,* Article ID: 770.

17. Vohs, K. D., & Baumeister, R. F. (Eds.). (2016). *Handbook of self-regulation: Research, theory, and applications.* New York: Guilford Press.

18. Menezes, C. B., Dalpiaz, N. R., Kiesow, L. G., Sperb, W., Hertzberg, J., & Oliveira, A. A. (2015). Yoga and emotion regulation: A review of primary psychological outcomes and their physiological correlates. *Psychology & Neuroscience,* 8(1), 82–101.

19. Faulds R. (2005). *Kripalu yoga: A guide to practice on and off the mat.* New York: Bantam Books.

20. Iyengar, B. K. S. (1966). *Light on yoga.* New York: Schocken Books.

21. Firestone, K., Carson, J., Mist, S., Carson, K., & Jones, K. (2014). Interest in yoga among fibromyalgia patients: An international internet survey. *International Journal of Yoga Therapy, 24,* 117–124.

22. Cramer, H., Lauche, R., Langhorst, J., & Dobos, G. (2013). Yoga for depression: A systematic review and meta-analysis. *Depression and Anxiety, 30,* 1068–1083.

23. National Center for Complementary and Integrative Health (NCCIH). (2017). Yoga: In depth | NCCIH. Retrieved on March 12, 2018, from https://nccih.nih.gov/health/yoga/introduction.htm#hed3

24. Lasater, J. H. (2016). *A year of living your yoga: Daily practices to shape your life.* Boulder, CO: Shambhala Publications.

25. Carlson, L. E., Speca, M., Faris, P., & Patel, K. D. (2007). One year pre–post intervention follow-up of psychological, immune, endocrine and blood pressure outcomes of mindfulness-based stress reduction (MBSR) in breast and prostate cancer outpatients. *Brain, Behavior, and Immunity, 21,* 1038–1049.

CHAPTER SEVEN

Yoga: Addressing Physical Functioning and Well-Being in Older Adults

T. Anne Richards and Angela DiMartino

> Yoga helps integrate the mental and the physical plane, and it offers a sense of inner and outer balance and alignment. True alignment means that the inner mind reaches every cell and fiber of the body.
>
> —B. K. S. Iyengar[1]

Yoga has been a healing tradition since it was first systematized and recorded by Patanjali (200 BCE) in the Yoga Sutras, 195 aphorisms mapping the philosophy and practice of yoga as a system intended to cease the fluctuations of the mind, bring peace to the experiences of daily life, and draw one into spiritual harmony. While schools of yoga or systems of practices vary, three of the components (or limbs) of yoga remain *asana* (physical poses), *pranayama* (breathing practices), and meditation (*dhyana* or focusing of attention). Yoga's use in direct medical applications began in 1918 near Mumbai, India, and since the 1970s, a number of studies, including clinical trials, have been conducted in both the West and the East examining the effects of yoga on a number of conditions, including psychopathologies, cardiovascular diseases, respiratory diseases, muscular-skeletal disorders, and metabolic disorders.[2] The growing number of exploratory studies and clinical trials has resulted in the use of yoga as both an alternative and adjunct treatment.

Older adults in the United States are increasingly living with multiple (two to four) chronic conditions (MCC). With the "graying" of the very sizable baby boomer generation and gen X now entering older adulthood, both seniors and health practitioners are looking to find ways of managing MCC. Yoga shows potential as a complementary therapy in the treatment of MCC. This chapter examines the impact of MCC in the aging process and yogic practices that have been shown to be effective in managing these conditions and, in turn, improving well-being.

Living in a Body

Like it or not, the physical body, the magnificent temple in which we dwell, is temporary. Over time, the body wears out or breaks down—sometimes slower, sometimes faster, sometimes painfully, sometimes suddenly and without warning. Factors such as genetics, lifestyle, socioeconomics, psychological and emotional conditions, and the environment all play a role in determining the course of health or illness for each individual. Meanwhile, our spirits call out to live our lives to the fullest, with as much meaning as possible, in whatever life circumstances we face.

Often, spiritual practices are resources for making peace with our temporal lives. Yoga is both a physical and meditative practice with the capability to harmonize what yoga considers our multiple bodies: the physical, the physiological or energetic, the mental-emotional, the intellectual/wisdom, and the blissful or source of fulfillment and joy.[1] When engaged, yoga can be a very practical, enjoyable, and beneficial practice for those moving into later years.

Resisting Medicalization of the Body and the Self

Medical care needs to be embraced as a practical engagement in dealing with chronic illness; yet we want to be recognized as more than a set of symptoms. It is well established that a "whole-person" approach is the better model for care.[3] Medical perspectives are shifting away from sole reliance on prescription-based management toward the advocacy of lifestyle changes incorporated into treatment plans. While support from health-care providers is wanted and needed, there is also an urgency to direct our own lives and bodies. This becomes increasingly true as we age. It is hard to come to grips with the aging body. It is hard to give up habits that may have contributed to the breaking down of our bodies. It is recognized that a collaborative approach between the person and the provider is a more productive relationship, taking into account what an individual might or might not do in order to improve health, well-being, and quality of life.[4] Approaches that integrate alternative and spiritual practices can be an important part of providers' "medical tool kit," particularly when caring for older adults with MCC.

Multiple Chronic Conditions among Older Adults

Background/ Prevalence

The United States is expected to experience significant growth in its older population through the aging of the baby boomers (born between 1946 and 1964) and generation X (born between 1965 and 1980) and increased life expectancy.[5] The number of people aged 65 and older is expected to double from 46 million (as of December 2015) to more than 98 million by 2060.[6] Gen X members will start turning 65 in 2030 and are projected to pass the baby boomer generation in size by 2028.[7] A recent survey comparing attitudes about health and longevity between gen X and baby boomers revealed that while gen X feels that their lifestyle choices play a great role in their health, they are less likely than baby boomers to take the necessary preventive health measures to maintain health.[8]

While having a single chronic condition, such as diabetes or high blood pressure, has negative health implications, MCC has an even greater impact on health. The risk of having more than one chronic condition increases with age; Vogeli and colleagues note that "62% of Americans over age 65 have MCC" (p. 392).[9] By 2020, 81 million Americans are projected to have MCC.[10] Of men and women aged 45 to 64, 28.1 percent have two or three MCC; this figure increases to 45.4 percent after age 65 for men and 47.4 percent for women.[11]

Research has shown that certain chronic conditions tend to cluster together. Arthritis and hypertension make up the top dyad of chronic conditions occurring in men (49.3 percent) and women (63 percent) over 65 years of age.[11] The top triad of MCC for men and women over 65 years of age is arthritis, diabetes, and hypertension (men = 28.2 percent, women = 32.6 percent). The age bracket below 65 (age 45 to 64) experience the same common dyads and triads of MCC at similar rates.[11] However, the prevalence of MCC in certain subgroups (women overall, black/African American men and women, American Indian men and women) is higher than in other subgroups.[11,12]

Importance

There are several reasons why finding interventions to treat chronic conditions of older adults is important. Having MCC leads to greater chances of developing comorbidities and increases premature mortality. A literature review of 41 articles about the impacts of MCC on aging showed there is a reduced quality of life, increased risk of disability, and hastened functional decline.[12] Each condition causes physiological changes. For example, arthritis can cause chronic pain, impaired mobility, and a reduction in the ability to do normal activities of life. Suffering from chronic pain and seeking help from medications can lead to the use of opioids, leading to greater risk of falls, heart disease, and accidental overdose.[13] Functional decline in the ability to handle the normal "activities of daily living" (ADLs; feeding, bathing, and dressing) can lead to the need for caregiver support and make it more difficult for one to remain independent in the home. Another major concern for those with MCC is being a "burden to their loved ones" (p. 55).[10]

One's body and mind are intrinsically intertwined. Compounding the impacts on the physical body, MCC also have negative impacts on emotional health and quality of life. A study of 15,000 patients showed that the poorest level of quality of life was found in patients who were older, female, and had at least one comorbid condition.[14] An international comparison study of self-reported quality of life of adults from eight countries showed that individuals with chronic conditions scored worse that those individuals without any chronic conditions.[15] Specifically, poorer quality of life outcomes were reported by those with cardiovascular conditions or diabetes.[16] A two-year longitudinal study noted that patients with chronic disease who had higher baseline physical activity had better functioning and well-being at baseline and two years later.[17] Helping patients manage their MCC may lead to improved quality of life and well-being.

Considering the top triad of conditions that cluster together (arthritis, diabetes, hypertension), risk factors of sedentary lifestyle, unhealthy eating habits, obesity, and chronic stress have all been implicated in the development of this triad of conditions.[18] When one suffers the pain of arthritis, exercising or even moving around becomes difficult. This often begins a circle of less physical activity leading to weight gain, causing more pain on already vulnerable joints. Diabetes and hypertension can develop and be exacerbated through poor eating habits, lack of exercise, and chronic stress. Yoga studies are providing growing evidence of health benefits for the three MCC of diabetes, arthritis, and hypertension and shows great promise as an adjunct therapy in management and treatment of these conditions.

Yoga: Physical Functioning and Well-Being

Part of the complexity in studying the effects of yoga is that there are many approaches to practices involving different schools, philosophies, and systems. It is difficult to get a consistent body of evidence-based interventions because of the variations of practices and methodologies for measuring yoga,[19] and this is readily pointed out in study limitations sections. That said, yoga research continues, and there is a growing body of evidence of the potential of yogic practices in managing chronic illnesses. An aspect that needs to be considered is that the practice and study of yoga varies in different cultures.[20] Taking cultural considerations into account, we keep an eye toward what is not only effective but practical and acceptable in the U.S. population of older adults, our target population, which has its own set of cultural and social variations.

The literature review on evidence-based yoga practices was focused on studies directed toward the three prevalent conditions of arthritis, hypertension, and diabetes. Not all interventions were focused on older adults, but most included adults over 60. Disability factors associated with each chronic disease were taken into consideration, and yoga interventions were designed in accordance with these limiting factors.

Hypertension

In a review and meta-analysis by Hagins, States, Selfe, and Innes, a preliminary recommendation was made for yoga as an intervention for hypertension based on pooled results from 17 studies.[21] Yoga was associated with significant decline in both systolic (p = 0.0002) and diastolic (p = 0.0001) blood pressure. Interventions using three elements of yoga (*asana, pranayama,* and meditation) showed the greatest impact, and results were of the greatest clinical and prognostic significance. The length of most U.S. interventions was between 6 and 12 weeks with one to three weekly sessions, 30 to 90 minutes in duration. Interventions in India were of longer duration, extending as long as 36 to 40 weeks.

Another review by Cramer and colleagues examined seven RCTs and viewed the evidence of impact on hypertension as "emerging but low quality" due principally to the quality of the research and variations of yoga styles and techniques.[22] In their meta-analysis, there were meaningful improvements in both systolic (p = 0.01) and diastolic (p = 0.02) blood pressure for those with hypertension. Breathing (*pranayama*) interventions showed greater effectiveness than those that were *asana* (poses) based. Yoga was found to be effective as an adjunct to medication but not as an alternative. U.S. interventions ranged from 6 to 12 weeks, with one to three sessions per week, 55 to 70 minutes in duration.

There are several types of *pranayama* practices, some involving slow breathing and others involving fast breathing. A study examining the effects of slow and fast breathing[23] on hypertension found slow breathing had the greater effect in decreasing blood pressure over a three-month period. The intervention involved daily sessions of *pranayama* for 15 minutes per session. Participants were trained in breathing techniques by a qualified instructor during the first week. Subsequently, participants practiced on their own with intermittent checks by trained instructors.

Arthritis

Haaz and Bartlett conducted a scoping review of 11 randomized controlled trials (RCT) and non-RCT trials, from 1980 through 2010, on effects of yoga on both rheumatoid arthritis (RA) and osteoarthritis (OA).[24] Study design and variations of yoga protocol interfered with the ability to draw conclusions across studies. Consistent clinical evidence was found for significant reduction in symptoms of tender/swollen joints and disability as well as improvements in mental health, self-efficacy, and energy in persons with RA. Significant decreases in pain were found in studies of both RA and OA. Levels of significance were not reported. Haaz and Bartlett noted that OA and RA are the most common diagnosis of arthritis but have "significant pathophysiologic differences" (pg. 8) and would most likely require different kinds of yoga interventions in order to be effective.[24]

Intervention protocols and styles of yoga varied, but most integrated *asana*, *pranayama*, meditation, and relaxation. Length of interventions ranged from 6 to 16 weeks with most lasting six to eight weeks. Sessions ranged from 40 to 150 minutes, with 60 or 90 minutes most common.

Most sessions were conducted once or twice per week, and some interventions incorporated home practices in addition to sessions taught by certified teachers. Yoga protocols were not described in all studies. However, several studies did indicate the use of modifications of yoga poses using props for support, chair yoga, and gentle yoga. One intervention was developed by a certified yoga therapist and a rheumatologist. Another was developed by registered yoga therapists, rheumatologists, and psychologists.

Following Haaz and Bartlett's (2011) scoping review, Moonaz, Bingham, Wissow, and Bartlett developed a randomized controlled pragmatic trial that tested the effectiveness of an intervention in a broad clinical practice, bridging the gap between research and care.[25] The trial evaluated the effects of integral-based hatha yoga on sedentary adults with RA or OA. Results showed significant improvements in walking capacity, vitality, and general health with decreases in pain and depression and increases in positive affect and quality of life ($p < 0.05$) measured at eight weeks. Intervention effects persisted when measured at nine months post intervention. The authors concluded that there was preliminary evidence that yoga could be effectively used for sedentary adults with arthritis, improving physical and psychological health.

The intervention used in this trial lasted eight weeks with two 60-minute classes and one home practice per week. Poses were modified according to individual needs. The system of yoga used, integral hatha yoga, includes the practices of *asana*, *pranayama*, and meditation. The intervention was designed by a registered yoga therapist in conjunction with faculty at Johns Hopkins Arthritis Center. Classes were taught by two yoga therapists trained in addressing diverse, specialized needs.

Sharma reviewed research conducted between 2010 and 2013 on the use of yoga for managing arthritis.[26] Nine articles met inclusion criteria—five from the United States and four from India. Limitations regarding study design and variations in yoga protocols were noted. Five of the nine studies showed varying statistically significant results in pain reduction and related disability. Based on the summary of evidence, the authors concluded that yoga was a "promising modality" (p. 51).[26]

Interventions conducted in the United States were of six to eight weeks in length with practices once or twice per week, 45 to 90 minutes in duration. Interventions in India were of longer duration. The author expressed the need for the development of a list of essential techniques that could be replicated and tested in future studies. Sharma also stated that the length of intervention and the number of practice sessions need to be easily embraced while still being long enough to be effective on a short- and long-term basis. It was suggested that interventions have both training and home practice components.

Diabetes

There is a high incidence of type 2 diabetes in India, and the majority of the studies found on yoga and diabetes were conducted in India. This has implications for the duration and intensity of yoga interventions for diabetes that were investigated. Yoga is more established as part of the Indian culture, and interventions tend to be long and intense, which are most likely beyond the capacity or acceptance of the U.S. population. Taking that into account, all results are still presented.

Thind and colleagues conducted a systematic review and meta-analysis of 23 studies to examine the effects of yoga on glycemic control in adults with type 2 diabetes.[27] Studies were conducted between 1991 and 2015. In the meta-analysis, yoga participants significantly improved their HbA1c ($p < 0.001$), fasting blood glucose (FBG) ($p < 0.001$), and postprandial blood sugar (PPBS), ($p = 0.025$). All aspects of the lipid profiles also showed significant reductions ($p < 0.001$). Long-term efficacy was not determined.

Interventions in this review used *asana* (96 percent), *pranayama*/breathing exercises (91 percent), relaxation techniques (70 percent), meditation (39 percent), and yogic philosophy (9 percent). Intervention lengths ranged from 1 to 26 weeks with numbers of sessions per week ranging from one to seven with an average duration of 60 minutes. Home practices were encouraged in 45 percent of the interventions.

In examining two individual studies not included in the Thind and colleagues' (2007) review, there was overlap in outcomes and types of yoga interventions with different intervention lengths (Bijlani et al., 2005; Singh, Kyizom, Singh, Tandon, & Madhu, 2008).[28,29] These studies found yoga to have similar levels of significant benefits in metabolic parameters and lipid profiles.

The intervention by Bijlani and colleagues found significant reductions in FBG ($p < 0.001$) and lipid profiles ($p < 0.001$).[28] HbA1c was not assessed. The program integrated theory and practice sessions that included *asana*, *pranayama*, meditation, and relaxation. Ninety-eight participants took part in training groups of six to eight participants. The program was an eight-day immersion (with a weekend break) led by expert instructors.

Singh and colleagues found significant reductions in FBG ($p < 0.001$), PPBS ($p < 0.001$), and lipid profiles ($p < 0.05$).[29] HbA1c was not assessed. This intervention lasted 45 days, 45 minutes per day, using *asana*, *pranayama*, and relaxation. The intervention was led by an expert instructor at the beginning, and then participants practiced on their own with follow-up calls from an instructor to support compliance. Long-term implications were unknown. The question was raised: To what degree does yoga practice need to be continued in order to sustain results?

Well-Being and Quality of Life

In the studies reviewed, only a few involved interventions that measured impact on well-being and quality of life. In Haaz and Bartlett's scoping review of arthritis interventions, psychosocial outcomes were examined in 7 of the 11 studies reviewed.[24] In five of the seven studies, improvements were found in affect, self-efficacy, emotional roles, depressive symptoms, vitality, and global mental health.

Moonaz and colleagues then went on to conduct a randomized controlled pragmatic trial to evaluate an integral-based yoga program in sedentary people with arthritis.[25] Integral yoga synthesizes various branches of yoga with the aim of developing harmony within the individual. In this style of yoga, there is a greater emphasis on spiritual aspects of yoga when compared with other styles more frequently used in research. Results of this trial showed significant improvements ($p < 0.05$) in positive affect, depression, self-efficacy, and most health-related quality-of-life domains at eight weeks, and effects were still evident at nine months post intervention.

Putting It Together

There was common ground across all studies and conditions reviewed. The combination of *asana*, *pranayama*, meditation, and relaxation were effective across the three conditions of hypertension, arthritis, and diabetes. Interventions were developed by expert trainers or yoga therapists, sometimes in conjunction with specialists such as rheumatologists or psychologists. Asana practices were often adapted for older populations or disabled populations, using gentle styles and supports of yoga props, chairs, and walls. Warm-ups to prepare for *asanas* were often incorporated and involved both gentle stretching and breathing. Trainings were conducted in groups of approximately 8 to 12 participants, all of whom had one or more diagnosis of a chronic condition. Groups were led by well-trained yoga experts or yoga therapists. Interventions in the United States typically lasted for 6 to 12 weeks. Sessions were typically 30 to 90 minutes in duration, conducted one to three times per week. Home practices were integrated into some interventions and recommended by several authors. Although recommended, the difficulty of sustaining home practices was noted. Often, the home practices that were used in the interventions were of short duration.

Multiple styles of yoga were used in the interventions, including Iyengar, integral, restorative, ashtanga, yoga nidra, vinyasana, and kundalini. Iyengar style yoga was most frequently used in the interventions, followed by integral yoga. Regardless of the style, there were certain *asana* and *pranayama* practices that were consistently incorporated into the interventions. *Asanas* include standing, seated, reclining, prone, and inversion poses, forward bends, backbends, twists, balancing poses, and poses for meditation and deep relaxation. Sequencing of *asanas* varied. Modifications and the use of props were applied on a case-by-case basis. The requirement for appropriate sequencing, modifications, and propping underscore the need for well-trained and experienced yoga instructors/therapists. Table 7.1 provides a list of *asanas* across interventions and conditions.

Asana practice is a gateway to *pranayama* and relaxation. *Pranayama* is regulated and controlled breathing, often involving interrupting the breath at certain intervals. There are a number of types of *pranayama*, some not suitable for beginners. Not all studies specified which types of *pranayama* were used, but the practices that prevailed were slow breathing practices with an emphasis on what can be called a "full-body breath" or "full yogic breath." These practices expand the entirety of the torso, using the lower abdominal muscles to act as something of a bellows, drawing the breath from deep in the torso and filling the torso to the top. Depending on the specific *pranayama* practice, the breath is controlled or interrupted in certain patterns. Of the practices named, *pranayama* that involved alternate nostril breathing was most prevalent (*nadi shuddhi*, *nadi sohana*, and *viloma*). These practices, particularly *nadi shuddhi* and *nadi sohana*, are acceptable practices for beginners.

Fast breathing practices were only specified in the diabetes interventions, most of which were conducted in India. The prevalent fast breathing practices were *bahastrika* (bellows breath), and *kapalbhati* (skull shining breath). Both of these practices are intermediate to advanced practices, and caution is warranted in introducing these practices to older American adults with MCC.

Meditation practices were not specifically defined. One study named the use of mindfulness meditation. Given the emphasis on *pranayama* in most studies, it might be inferred that meditation practices were centered on attention to the breath. However, this was not explicitly stated.

Table 7.1   Asanas Used in Interventions

Sanskrit	English
Poses consistently used:	
Tadasana (always used)	Mountain pose (standing)
Trikonasana	Triangle pose (standing)
Paschimottanasana	Forward bend (seated)
Surya Namaskar	Sun Salutation (standing series)
Savasana (always used)	Corpse pose (reclining)
Poses often used:	
Bhujangasana	Cobra pose (prone backbend)
Shalabasana	Locust pose (prone backbend)
Dhanurasana	Bow pose (prone backbend)
Vajrasana	Thunderbolt pose (seated, kneeling)
Vrikshasana	Tree pose (standing, balance)
Konasana	Side angle pose (standing)
Utthita Padmasana	Straight leg raising pose (reclining)
Pavanamuktasana	Wind releasing pose (reclining)
Setu Bandhasana	Bridge pose (reclining)
Virabhadrasana I, II, III	Warrior poses (standing)
Dandasana	Staff pose (seated)
Other poses used:	
Ardhakati Chakrasana	Lateral arc pose (standing)
Uttanasana	Forward bend (standing)
Makarasana	Crocodile pose (prone)
Sarvangasana	Shoulder stand (inversion)
Matsyasana	Fish pose (reclining back bend)
Baddha Konasana	Bound angle pose (seated)
Ardha Matsyendrasana	Half spinal twist (seated)
Sarpasana	Snake pose (prone backbend)
Supta Padangusthasana	Hand to big toe pose (reclining)
Supta Tadasana	Mountain pose (reclining)
Urdhva Hastasana	Raised hands pose (standing)
Ardha Uttanasana	Half forward bend (standing)
Adho Mukha Svanasana	Downward dog pose (standing)
Padmasana or Sukhasana	Lotus or Easy pose (cross legged seated)

What is referred to as "relaxation" in yoga most typically means the practice of *savasana* (corpse pose), which is done as the last asana of any class. In some classes, particularly restorative yoga, *savasana* will be done at both the beginning and end of class. It is a reclining pose that can be propped in a number of ways and is intended, at the end of class, to allow the mind to quiet and focus inward and the body to completely relax and integrate the work of the class.

Delivering Interventions

There are practical issues to consider when thinking about yoga as an adjunct therapy for older adults with MCC. Medical practices, clinics, HMOs, or other health-care facilities or senior centers with an orientation toward patient-centered care would show the greatest promise for the introduction of yoga as complementary care. Within these locations, it is possible to gain collaboration of multidisciplinary teams working with the prevalent MCCs in their patient population. These locations would also have the ability to perform outreach for recruitment and retention. They have the capacity to offer an intervention series, track improvements in health, and offer maintenance classes to those who complete the initial intervention series.

In order for yoga to be effective in the treatment of MCC, it most likely needs to become a part of daily life. Group practices offer social engagement and support from peers while providing expert training in *asana*, *pranayama*, and relaxation. While it is difficult to cultivate engagement in home practices, peer support and training in catching "moments of yoga" (i.e., minipractices) throughout the day has the possibility of creating lifestyle change that might in turn change the quality of the day and improve physical health and overall well-being.

References

1. Iyengar, B. K. S. (1993). *Light on the yoga sutras*. London, England: Aquarian Press/HarperCollins.

2. Richards, T. A. (2010). The path of yoga. In T. G. Plante (Ed.), *Contemplative practices in action: Spirituality, meditation and health* (pp. 143–158). Santa Barbara, CA: Praeger.

3. Mean, N., & Bower, P. (2000). Patient-centeredness: A conceptual framework and review of the empirical literature. *Social Science and Medicine, 51*(7), 1087–1110. https://doi.org/10.1016/S0277-9536(00)00098-8

4. Frantsve, L. M. E., & Kerns, R. D. (2007). Patient–provider interactions in the management of chronic pain: Current findings within the context of shared medical decision making. *Pain Medicine, 8,* 25–35. doi:10.1111/j.1526-4637.2007.00250.x

5. United States Census Bureau. (2014). *An aging nation: The older population in the United States*. Retrieved on March 12, 2018, from https://www.census .gov/prod/2014pubs/p25-1140.pdf

6. Mather, M., Jacobsen, L. A., & Pollard, K. M. (2015). Aging in the United States. *Population Bulletin, 70*(2), 1–23.

7. Fry, R. (2016, April 25). Millennials overtake baby boomers as America's largest generation. *Pew Research Center*. Retrieved on March 12, 2018, from http://www.pewresearch.org/fact-tank/2016/04/25/millennials-overtake-baby -boomers///

8. Klemes, A. (2017, January 29). Gen X: The time to get serious about longevity is now. *MDVIP*. Retrieved on March 12, 2018, from https://www.mdvip .com/about-mdvip/blog/gen-x-time-to-get-serious-about-longevity

9. Vogeli, C., Shields, A. E., Lee, T. A., Gibson, T. B., Marder, W. D., Weiss, K. B., & Blumenthal, D. (2007). Multiple chronic conditions: Prevalence, health consequences, and implications for quality, care management, and costs. *Journal of General Internal Medicine, 22*(Suppl 3), 391–395. doi:10.1007/s11606-007 -0322-1

10. Partnership for Solutions. (2004). *Chronic conditions: Making the case for ongoing care*. Retrieved on March 12, 2018, from https://www.rwjf.org/en/library /research/2004/09/chronic-conditions-.html

11. Ward, B. W., & Schiller, J. S. (2013). Prevalence of multiple chronic conditions among US adults: Estimates from the National Health Interview Survey, 2010. *Preventing Chronic Disease, 10,* 1–15. http://dx.doi.org/10.5888/pcd10 .120203

12. Marengoni, A., Angleman, S., Melis, R., Mangialasche, F., Karp, A., Garmen, A., . . . Fratiglioni, L. (2011). Aging with multimorbidity: A systematic review of the literature. *Ageing Research Reviews, 10*(4), 430–439. http://dx.doi .org/10.1016/j.arr.2011.03.003

13. Dowell, D., Haegerich, T. M., & Chou, R. (2016). CDC guideline for prescribing opioids for chronic pain—United States, 2016. *JAMA, 315*(15), 1624– 1645. doi:10.1001/jama.2016.1464

14. Sprangers, M. A. G., deRegt, E. B., Andries, F., vanAgt, H. M. E., Bijl, R. E., deBoer, J. B., & deHaes, H. C. J. M. (2000). Which chronic conditions are associated with better or poorer quality of life? *Journal of Clinical Epidemiology, 53*(9), 895–907. https://doi.org/10.1016/S0895-4356(00)00204-3

15. Alonso, J., Ferrer, M., Gandek, B., Ware, J. E., Jr., Aaronson, N. K., Mosconi, P., & Leplège, A. (2004). Health-related quality of life associated with chronic conditions in eight countries: Results from the International Quality of Life Assessment (IQLA) Project. *Quality of Life Research, 13*(2), 283–298. https:// doi.org/10.1023/B:QURE.0000018472.46236.05

16. Chen, H.-Y., Baumgardner, D. J., & Rice, J. P. (2011). Health-related quality of life among adults with multiple chronic conditions in the United States, Behavioral Risk Factor Surveillance System, 2007. *Preventing Chronic Disease, 8*(1), A09.

17. Stewart, A. L., Hays, R. D., Wells, K. B., Rogers, W. H., Spritzer, K. L., & Greenfield, S. (1994). Long-term functioning and well-being outcomes associated with physical activity and exercise in patients with chronic conditions in the medical outcomes study. *Journal of Clinical Epidemiology, 47*(7), 719–730. https://doi.org/10.1016/0895-4356(94)90169-4

18. U.S. Department of Health and Human Services, Centers for Disease Control and Prevention. (2015). *Four domains of chronic disease prevention.* Retrieved on March 12, 2018, from https://www.cdc.gov/chronicdisease/resources/publications/four-domains.htm

19. Cohen, V. S., & Adams, T. B. (2005). Physical and perceptual benefits of yoga asana practice: Results of a pilot study. *Journal of Bodywork and Movement Therapies, 9,* 211–219.

20. Innes, K. E., & Vincent, H. K. (2007). The influence of yoga-based programs on risk profiles in adults with type 2 diabetes mellitus: A systematic review. *Evidence-Based Complementary and Alternative Medicine, 4*(4), 469–486. doi:10.1093/ecam/nel103

21. Hagins, M., States, R., Selfe, T., & Innes, K. (2013). Effectiveness of yoga for hypertension: Systematic review and meta-analysis. *Evidence-Based Complementary and Alternative Medicine, 2013*(649836), 1–13. http://dx.doi.org/10.1155/2013/649836

22. Cramer, H., Haller, H., Lauche, R., Steckhan, N., Michalsen, A., & Dobos, G. (2014). A systematic review and meta-analysis of yoga for hypertension. *American Journal of Hypertension, 27*(9), 1146–1151. https://doi.org/10.1093/ajh/hpu078

23. Mourya, M., Mahajan, A. S., Singh, N. P., & Jain, A. K. (2009). Effects of slow- and fast-breathing exercises on autonomic functions in patients with essential hypertension. *Journal of Alternative and Complementary Medicine, 15*(7), 711–717. https://doi.org/10.1089/acm.2008.0609

24. Haaz, S., & Bartlett, S. J. (2011). Yoga for arthritis: A scoping review. *Rheumatic Disease Clinics of North America, 37*(1), 33–46. https://doi.org/10.1016/j.rdc.2010.11.00111

25. Moonaz, S., Bingham III, C. O., Wissow, L., & Bartlett, S. J. (2015). Yoga in sedentary adults with arthritis: Effects of a randomized controlled pragmatic trial. *Journal of Rheumatology, 42*(7), 1194–1202. https://doi.org/10.3899/jrheum.141129

26. Sharma, M. (2014). Yoga as an alternative and complementary approach for arthritis: A systematic review. *Journal of Evidence-Based Complementary and Alternative Medicine, 19*(1), 51–58. https://doi.org/10.1177/2156587213499918

27. Thind, H., Lantini, R., Balletto, B. L., Donahue, M. L., Salmoirago-Blotcher, E., Bock, B. C., & Scott-Sheldon, L. A. J. (2017). The effects of yoga among adults with type 2 diabetes: A systematic review and meta-analysis. *Preventive Medicine, 105,* 116–126. https://doi.org/10.1016/j.ypmed.2017.08.017

28.   Bijlani, R. L., Vempati, R. P., Yadav, R. K., Ray, R. B., Gupta, V., Sharma, R., . . . Mahapatra, S. C. (2005). A brief from comprehensive lifestyle education program based on yoga reduces risk factors for cardiovascular disease and

diabetes mellitus. *Journal of Alternative and Complementary Medicine, 11*(2), 267–274. https://doi.org/10.1089/acm.2005.11.267

29. Singh, S., Kyizom, T., Singh, K. P., Tandon, O. P., & Madhu, S. V. (2008). Influence of pranayamas and yoga-asanas on serum insulin, blood glucose and lipid profile in type 2 diabetes. *Indian Journal of Clinical Biochemistry, 23*(4), 365–368. https://doi.org/10.1007/s12291-08-0080-9

Spiritual Models: Reflecting on *The Way of a Pilgrim* with Postsecondary Students at Risk of Stress, Depression, and Anxiety

*Suzette Brémault-Phillips, Ashley Pike,
and Joanne K. Olson*

Young Adulthood as a Time of Vulnerability and Spiritual Growth

Postsecondary student life can be a double-edged sword. Students are offered many opportunities for discovery, learning, and personal growth that can effectively prime them for successful lifelong pursuits. Many believe that their education will afford them a range of employment opportunities and ensure financial success. During their years of university education, students may also look forward to meeting new people, exploring their identity, and becoming increasingly independent.[1] Simultaneously, the transition to university and adulthood can also be stressful due to societal, social, academic, parental, and financial pressures. In this period of significant transition, social instability and identity crises can easily arise.[2] Preexisting or newly developing mental health conditions can make postsecondary life even more challenging.

Evidence indicates that many postsecondary students struggle with mental health issues and substance use.[3] Worldwide, half of mental illnesses begin by age 14, and three-quarters by the midtwenties.[4] In Canada, 15–24-year-olds have the highest incidence of mental disorders.[5] A National College Health Assessment conducted in 2016 among postsecondary students 18 to 30+ years of age across Canada and the United States found that, within a period of 12 months, students reported feeling so depressed that it was difficult for them to function (44.4 percent and 36.7 percent, respectively); felt things were hopeless (59.6 percent and 49.8 percent); seriously considered suicide (13.0 percent and 9.8 percent); and identified stress (42.2 percent and 33.8 percent), anxiety (32.5 percent and 23.2 percent), sleep (28.4 percent and 20.7 percent), and depression (20.9 percent and 15.4 percent) as the top factors affecting academic performance.[6,7] Regrettably, postsecondary students are also the least likely to seek help.[8]

Well-Being and Resilience among Postsecondary Students

Increasing emphasis has been placed on student mental health as more postsecondary students experience challenges, seek help, and present with complex issues. Heightened awareness of mental health as a key dimension of student life and its impact on learning, academic success, and overall well-being has become a priority for colleges and universities.[3] Internationally, trends supporting mental health and well-being have focused on the recovery model, child and youth mental health, and the role of schools, including postsecondary institutions.[3] In 2013, the Canadian Association of College and University Student Services produced a whitepaper entitled "Post-Secondary Student Mental Health: Guide to a Systemic Approach" (PSSMH)[9] with the aim of enabling student mental health to flourish rather than languish. In the PSSMH, institutions are seen as having the privilege and ethical responsibility to provide a range of services, resources, and supports that guide students through their academic careers and equip them with skills to thrive as citizens. Service provision at three levels of engagement are outlined, including at the campus community level, the individual student level (training in coping, resilience, and self-management skills), and the mental health service-delivery level. It is hoped that academic success, well-being, and mental health will be promoted through these activities.

Case Study: Undergraduate Practical Theology Course

To support student resilience and mental health, an introductory practical theology course was introduced at a Canadian postsecondary institution. The course engaged psychological and spiritual wisdom and practices that cultivate well-being, resilience, and mental and spiritual health. Aligned with the PSSMH, the course created an inclusive and collaborative learning environment; heightened student awareness of well-being, resilience, and mental and spiritual health; introduced coping and resiliency skills; and encouraged self-management. A spiritual model—the pilgrim in a spiritual classic, *The Way of a Pilgrim*[10]—was integrated into the course as a means for students to reflect on the subject matter.

Spiritual Models Can Inspire and Guide

Throughout history, spiritual and religious traditions have emphasized the value of learning from and emulating the example of good or holy persons.[11-14] Found in all faith traditions, spiritual models inform people about how to choose wisely, self-regulate,[12] and live better, more virtuous lives.[15] Examples of spiritual models include Jesus, Buddha, Mohammed, Mohandas Gandhi, Mother Teresa, Billy Graham, Martin Luther King Jr., religious or spiritual leaders, family members, friends, and colleagues. Models observed through written media can also support learning[12] (e.g., the pilgrim in *The Way of a Pilgrim*).

As much of human learning is social, learning from individuals who demonstrate desirable characteristics, as well as patterns of thinking, behaving, and relating, is a powerful way to activate, acquire, and sustain beliefs, attitudes, and behaviors.[11,12,15-19] Those who want to deepen their understanding of spirituality or religion in fact often learn by observing others.[12,19] According to Bandura's social cognitive theory,[16] modeling influences can serve as "instructors, inhibitors, disinhibitors, facilitators, stimulus enhancers, and emotion arousers" (p. 50).[16] Such learning, identified by Bandura as observational learning, enables people to efficiently and safely develop behaviors and skills and avoid trial and error.[12]

Spiritual modeling includes four psychological processes that parallel observational learning.[12,14] *Attention* relates to the need to attend to the model's behavior; *retention* refers to remembering the behavior of interest; *reproduction* involves engaging in similar behaviors as the model; and *motivation* relates to the desire to behave like the model.[15] Knowledge about the likely risks and benefits of different courses of action can be gained vicariously by observing the attitudes and experiences of models.[16] Reflecting on the character of the pilgrim presents students with such a learning opportunity.

Description of *The Way of a Pilgrim*

The Way of a Pilgrim is an Eastern Christian spiritual classic set in 19th-century Russia. An easily read guidebook to the spiritual journey, it is one of the most influential spiritual books of the last hundred years. The text is a compilation of four tales that depict a poor, lame man's outward pilgrimage, his inner journey in his mind and heart, and his relationship with God. His encounters with people, various life events, and a spiritual way of life are described. Considered to be the most popular book on Eastern Christian spirituality available to an English-speaking readership, it has inspired people from every walk of life to embark upon a spiritual path.[20–22]

Believed to have been penned as a theological and literary text by one or several educated churchmen, the tales introduce various aspects of an Eastern Christian way of life. These include *hesychasm* (i.e., a mystical form of spirituality that the pilgrim practices and that permeates every aspect of his life), ceaseless prayer (i.e., being mindful of the constant presence of and one's relationship with God, and praying the Jesus Prayer: "Lord Jesus Christ, Son of God, have mercy on me, a sinner"), the *philokalia*[23] (i.e., a collection of spiritual texts written between the 4th and 15th centuries by spiritual masters and read by the pilgrim), and other spiritual practices (e.g., silence, stillness, breathing, walking, fasting, forgiveness, custody of the eye and heart, gratitude, compassion, study, spiritual direction, participation in the sacraments) that enable him to grow in virtue, humility, wisdom, and holiness.

The character of the pilgrim offers students an example of a spiritual model. By observing his life, they are introduced to means by which to grow in virtue and reach one's potential. The ordinariness of his story speaks to the possibility for everyone to likewise become all they can be. His earnest search for what is most important to him, desire to learn from spiritual models and life experiences, engagement in a spiritual way of life, and growth in character and virtue beckons readers to mindfully grow into the fullness of their own being with every breath and step.

The Spiritual Model of the Pilgrim: Highlights of Student Observational Learning

As a way of exploring what students learned by reading *The Way of a Pilgrim*, a qualitative secondary analysis was undertaken of written submissions by 92 undergraduate students enrolled in the course between 2015 and 2017. Submissions included three papers from each student. The first focused on myths of happiness (e.g., "I'll only be happy if or when . . . "), including consequences of, and alternatives to, believing the myth. The second paper was a character sketch of the pilgrim (including factors affecting his well-being and spiritual health). The third paper considered spiritual practices in which the pilgrim engaged. The final section of each paper focused on application to postsecondary student life regarding well-being and spiritual health.

Preliminary Findings

Preliminary findings suggest that reading *The Way of a Pilgrim* and reflecting on the main character were universally helpful. Students described the book as a "great tool for university students." One student wrote about being "incredibly influenced by this book. To take what is subtly taught and apply it to the journey of a modern day student—most would find that it is extremely relevant." Though written in a different time and context, the text remained "relatable to students as many of them are still trying to figure out who they are."

Students drew from the text what they found applicable. "Though it is difficult for students to live like hermits, they can assume a life of modesty and humility," practice unceasing prayer, and apply simple lessons such as "don't be overly attached to earthly possessions" or "be kind to others." They also appreciated that they, much like the pilgrim, are "searching for something" and want to "better understand who they are and their end goal in life." They recognized that their current journey, which has them "explore concepts, theories and utilize this knowledge to become the people that they are meant to become, is pivotal." They were also cognizant that "an obsessive pursuit of worldly belongings does not bring happiness." Indeed, *The Way of a Pilgrim* may "serve as a lesson to search for happiness in the right places."

Several broad themes emerged in the students' writings, including learning by observing a spiritual model; growth in self-awareness; the potency and responsibility of personal choices; perseverance and discipline; shifting perspectives; social connections; love of others; connecting with spirituality and God by engaging in spiritual practices (prayer, forgiveness, humility, gratitude, hope, perseverance); finding inner peace; facing and overcoming stress, anxiety, and depression; posttraumatic growth; and resilience. A description of these themes follows.

Learning by Observing the Pilgrim

Like the pilgrim, who listened to his grandfather about the ways of God and how to be a man of character, students benefitted from the pilgrim's experience. While a few students struggled to connect with the story, were skeptical of or turned off by the text's religious motifs, or required time to "understand the underlying wisdom of the work," they also appreciated that "there is wisdom in it and lessons to be learned." Students suggested that it would benefit most people to "integrate a certain degree of the pilgrim's way of life into their own."

Growth in Self-Awareness

This spiritual classic helped students recognize the importance of and need for reflection and self-awareness. "To calm oneself, mentally relax, and contemplate the inner desires and workings of your heart and spirit; this is the effect that *The Way of a Pilgrim* can have." The text taught them about values and the meaning of "learning to love yourself, to find unconditional love in God and those around us." Some took time to deeply reflect on their past experiences and who they desired to become. "I thought about what I had done, realized I had never acted so carelessly and impulsively, and recognized that I did not want to be the angry person I seemed to be becoming." They considered their choices and garnered insight into how to "live a more virtuous life through lessons learned in *The Way of a Pilgrim*." They recognized that they too can choose to either "cultivate a new way of thinking, or not. In the end, like the pilgrim, it all comes down to a person's attitude and choice."

Choices: Potency and Responsibility

Students embraced the potency and responsibility of their own free will in new ways. They noted that it is essential to "take control of our lives and actions, as the pilgrim has done." This highlighted the importance of engagement in intentional activities and practices that cultivate character: "I have learned so much and it has definitely helped me as a student. Although there have been times in my life that have been stressful (with school, work, and volunteering, I wanted to give up), I pushed myself by using intentional activity." Students noted being more aware of their choices and the impact of their choices on themselves and others.

Perseverance and Discipline

Though often meek, the pilgrim models determination, discipline, perseverance in hardships, and "remaining hopeful and motivated toward one's primary goals and objectives." Students were impressed by his level of commitment toward his desires, noting that it is "nothing short of inspiring" and "strongly speaks to students." They surmised that if they chose to use the same determination in their studies, they would more likely excel, and they were mindful that how one "pushes beyond adversity in search of goals is what defines us."

Shifting Perspectives

In reading the text, students related that they had "gained a new way of looking at the world" that helped them "shift perspective." They noted that the text both encouraged them to be more positive and reminded them that they have a lifetime to learn. Students highlighted the way in which the pilgrim teaches us that "gratitude, respect, honesty and virtues are key to everlasting happiness" and to "appreciate life, because it can change in any moment for better or worse." Some realized that "happiness comes from within" and by "appreciating the little things" that are often overlooked or taken for granted.

Social Connections

Reading *The Way of a Pilgrim* impressed upon students that "human inter-action is crucial to growth." While they might feel alone, there are many other people on the same journey. Reading the text encouraged them to con-sider who they spend time with, mindful that who one associates with reflects on who they are and become. It further challenged them to spend more time and energy on family, friends, and things that they love doing. Much as the pilgrim did, they felt that they may want to "cultivate brotherly love and seek mutual support." They concluded that it is important to "appre-ciate people in our lives," "learn from others," and listen, as "everybody has a different story."

Love of Others

Students recognized that, ultimately, this book "teaches us to be kind and compassionate to everyone. It is a worthwhile practice on a 21st century campus. To be loving, kind, and warmhearted is not only the foundation of healthy social practices, but of a healthy life." His journey and transformation is "an example and model of what students can do to become more compas-sionate and live happy and meaningful lives." As a spiritual model, his "acts of charity may inspire students to practice charity." They noted that "if we all lend a helping hand, we could make each other's journeys a little bit easier." They delighted in the fact that it "really doesn't take much to make someone smile, show compassion and love a neighbour."

Connection with Spirituality and God by Engaging in Spiritual Practices

Regarding spirituality, students described *The Way of a Pilgrim* as "a fan-tastic text for those seeking answers regarding their purpose" and reflecting on the importance of being spiritually healthy. They indicated that the book taught them to "have faith, find a passion and devote their life to it." Students were respectful that each person "has their own set of beliefs." Interestingly, they also noted that, while "some individuals may not be religious, *The Way of a Pilgrim* can still be read as an optimistic text that highlights the impor-tance of being connected to the spirit."

For those who believe in God, they indicated that reading this text may help people feel more connected to their faith, and insights from the text can be utilized to help them grow and deepen their relationship with God. They recognized that, while the pilgrim spent most of his time alone, he was never really alone, and nor are they. It reassured and comforted them that "while people come and go, God will always be with us." Students indicated that it would be helpful to remember this. Further, just as the pilgrim cultivated his relationship with God in order to be better able to give unconditional love and overcome tough moments, they can as well. They viewed doing so as contributing to well-being. "Having faith in something or opening up spiritually can have positive effects." By strengthening their relationship with God, they anticipated that they might be better able to manage the ups and downs of life.

Prayer

From the pilgrim's example, students learned that prayer is "continual union with God, and harmony of the body, mind, and heart" and saw it as "a powerful tool." They closely observed the pilgrim, who, after a life of tragedy and heartbreak, turned to prayer to find joy and happiness in his everyday life. His ability to find solace in praying unceasingly "contributed to his ability to manage his difficult circumstances." Students considered that practicing techniques such as the Jesus prayer might help them as well to "find peace, joy, and well-being." They observed how engaging in prayer and mindfulness can give one "a positive worldview, as well as joy and hope for the future."

Students considered prayer in the context of the overwhelming and stressful experience of academic life. They thought it important to look at how the pilgrim handled stress through prayer. "Praying can help an individual calm down, overcome stresses, and function better." They recognized the importance of "stopping the mind from wandering, and focusing on the present and what the heart desires." Students thought it possible to practice prayer by "mimicking the pilgrim's use of breathing, prayer, meditation, or affirmations," which they anticipated could support "growth in self-compassion, confidence, and connection to one's true self." By cultivating spiritual well-being, students indicated that they would be able to "develop healthy perspectives and cultivate happiness in their darkest times." Students also appreciated that spiritual well-being is achieved by "surrounding oneself with other believers who are of a similar mind-set." Like the pilgrim, who constantly sought mentorship and connection with believers, students indicated that it may be helpful for them to do the same.

Forgiveness and Humility

The pilgrim's example of forgiveness and humility also caught students' attention. They felt that by cultivating forgiveness and humility, they might be less depressed, happier, and healthier. Students considered ways in which the pilgrim teaches the reader through his words, actions, and relationships that the more appropriate response to a frustrating or hurtful situation is humility, "that much comes from forgiveness, and that nothing good comes from harboring envy or hatred." The pilgrim's ability to refrain from anger by being humble and gentle was notable to them, with students commenting that it is only "through humility, that we are able to forgive those who have wronged or hurt us," including our very selves.

Gratitude

Students felt that they could learn much from the pilgrim's "expression of gratitude which helped him heal from depression and grow in hope." They noted that the pilgrim was always grateful to people who showed kindness by providing for his physical or spiritual needs. Students found inspiration in his attitude of joy and thanksgiving regardless of the situation and appreciation for what he had as a way of overcoming negative turns of fortune. They considered how being grateful can open one's eyes to the smallest of small things and noted that gratitude can enable a person to embrace hope.

Hope

Students saw the pilgrim as a model whose "hope was radiant." It never ceased to amaze them that the "pilgrim never lost hope." Given the pilgrim's ability to find hope amid his life circumstances, they came to believe that hope is possible for everyone. They commented on the importance of looking toward and being optimistic about the future and not being "overcome by badness in the world." Appreciating the potency of hope, they noted that it is what helps them get through some days.

Perseverance through Struggles

Maintaining hope is particularly important in times of struggle. Students noted that the pilgrim's strength and perseverance even in the face of tragedies and adversities can be an inspiration to those struggling with papers and studying for exams. The pilgrim is an example of how "to appreciate good and bad events." His journey offers students guidance and reassurance, courage to brace against calamities, and encouragement that they can endure anything that comes their way. They noted that, while life can be full of trials, and events may be out of our control or self-inflicted, "our attitudes, actions, practices, and beliefs can heavily impact how we face hardships. Happiness is in our hands." One student noted that "it is beautiful observing an individual overcome past traumas and be transformed to a happier individual who is then able to help in the transformation of others."

Finding Inner Peace

Students felt that "one of the most important things we can learn from the pilgrim is to find inner peace." Students were impressed that, despite his upsetting early life, the pilgrim was able to find peace. They believed that they can do the same. "If a student is able to find peace, and joy, then they will be able to face any challenge." By reflecting on the pilgrim's life, students recognized that they can choose to use any number of practices to overcome struggles. They recognized the importance of "learning to look at life circumstances as opportunities for growth and focusing on the inner self and the present" as a way to find happiness even in times of darkness. They were inspired by the pilgrim's ability to celebrate what was beautiful in life, regardless of the circumstance.

Facing and Overcoming Stress, Anxiety, and Depression

The pilgrim provides a potent spiritual model for students in need of guidance in managing stress and anxiety or coping with depression and spiritual sadness. They indicated that reflecting on *The Way of a Pilgrim* offered them numerous significant insights. Like the pilgrim, when they find themselves grief-stricken, anxious, or angry, students may feel that "isolating themselves is the best way to heal." Despite this urge, they felt it important for students, like the pilgrim, to engage in social relationships. They also related that students can benefit from cultivating trusting relationships with people who both hold them accountable and support them in their journeys. Students also noted that it is important for them to not be afraid to ask for guidance and comfort—or help from parents, families, and God—during crucial moments.

Posttraumatic Growth

Students recognized that negative situations and circumstances can have a positive effect on one's life depending on how a person deals with them. They marveled that, despite having experienced so many negative events, the pilgrim never let these experiences hold him back; rather, he found a way to make them positive. Applying this lesson to their own lives, they noted that such events either define a person or help one grow. "It's all about perspective."

Resilience

Time and again, the pilgrim struggled through challenges but always picked himself up and continued on his journey. He is resilient. Students speculated that building resilience like the pilgrim would help them "bounce back and be successful." They felt that they could learn from him to "make intentional choices and find strength and resilience in engaging in spiritual practices." They recognize that, through such engagement, he "cultivated joy and resilience, which in turn helped him manage stress and sadness." Students suggested that the pilgrim illustrates "tremendous resilience after losing people closest to him, and facing many challenges along his journey." They found his example of resilience and perseverance to be applicable to anyone who experiences misfortunes. Students appreciated that "the more a person grows, learns and experiences, the more resilient to adverse situations they may be in the future."

Conclusion

Postsecondary institutions are important environments for promoting well-being, resilience, and mental and spiritual health. There is evidence indicating that students learn by observation, including of spiritual models found in literary and spiritual texts, such as *The Way of a Pilgrim*. A figure such as the pilgrim was found to act as an instructor, (dis)inhibitor, facilitator, stimulus enhancer, and emotion arouser.[16]

Conducting this secondary analysis enabled the authors to examine what students had learned about well-being, resilience, happiness, and mental and spiritual health by reflecting on a spiritual model in a literary and spiritual text. The psychological processes they underwent in reading about and reflecting on the pilgrim were in keeping with Bandura's observational learning. Students *attended* to and *remembered* the pilgrim's behavior, *mimicked* him, and were *motivated* to adopt something from his way of life. By observing his attitudes and experiences, they vicariously gained knowledge and insights. Students learned about spirituality and spiritual practices as means of personal growth; coping with stress, hardship, and struggle; being resilient; and reaching their potential. They also witnessed the transformative effects of practicing a spiritual way of life. By observation, they developed behaviors and skills and were transformed. From the student perspective, the pilgrim's journey gave them "a positive example to refer to in times of joy and struggle. His journey ultimately led him to be more virtuous and Christlike. A student's journey can also lead them to reach their full potential."

Based on study findings, it would be advantageous for students to be introduced to various spiritual models that can inspire them by their exemplary ways of life. This would provide them with models of citizenship, virtuous living, resilience, and well-being. Without examples, they can potentially be left floundering at a time when stresses are significant, and they are at risk of developing depression and anxiety. Fundamentally, students who have a sense of what is involved in a spiritual way of life and what is important to them are better equipped to maintain well-being, resilience, and mental and spiritual health, as well as manage challenges to their own mental health if they arise. They are also more clear about their own way of life and empowered to makes choices in keeping with it. As a result, they are better able to develop their character, foster well-being, reach their potential, be compassionate toward others, and contribute to the creation of a better world.

References

1. Arnett, J. J. (2014). Emerging adulthood: The winding road from the late teens through the twenties. *Oxford Scholarship Online.* doi:10.1093/acprof: oso/9780199929382.003.0006

2. Arnett, J. J., & Tanner, J. L. (2006). *Emerging adults in America: Coming of age in the 21st century.* Washington, DC: American Psychological Association.

3. MacKean, G. (2011). Mental health and well-being in post-secondary education settings. A literature and environmental scan to support planning and action in Canada. Retrieved on March 12, 2018, from http://campusmental health.ca/wpcontent/uploads/2014/02/Post_Sec_Final_Report_June6.pdf

4. World Health Organization. (2013). Mental health action plan 2013–2020. Retrieved on March 12, 2018, from http://apps.who.int/iris/bitstream/10665/89966 /1/9789241506021_eng.pdf?ua=1

5. Pearson, C., Janz, T., & Ali, J. (2013). *Health at a glance: Mental and substance use disorders in Canada.* Ottawa, ON: Statistics Canada. Retrieved on March 12, 2018, from http://www.statcan.gc.ca/pub/82-624-x/2013001/article /11855-eng.pdf

6. American College Health Association. (2016). *National College Health Assessment II: Canadian reference group executive summary, Spring 2016.* Hanover, MD: American College Health Association. Retrieved from http://www.cacuss .ca/_Library/Provincial_Reports/NCHA-II_SPRING_2016_CANADIAN_ REFERENCE_GROUP_EXECUTIVE_SUMMARY.pdf (link no longer active)

7. American College Health Association. (2016). *National College Health Assessment II: Reference group executive summary, Spring 2016.* Hanover, MD: American College Health Association. Retrieved on March 12, 2018, from http:// www.acha-ncha.org/docs/NCHA-II%20SPRING%202016%20US%20REFER ENCE%20GROUP%20EXECUTIVE%20SUMMARY.pdf

8. Everall, R. (2013). Student mental health at the University of Alberta. Final report of provost fellow. Edmonton, AB. Retrieved on March 12, 2018, from http://www.provost.ualberta.ca/en/~/media/provost/Documents/Information /SMHFull.pdf

9. Canadian Association of College and University Student Services (CACUSS). (2013). *Post-secondary student mental health: Guide to a systemic approach.* Vancouver, BC: Author. Retrieved from http://www.cacuss.ca/_Library /PSSMH/PSSMH_GuideToSystemicApproach_CACUSSCMHA_2013.pdf (link no longer active)

10. Pentkovsky, A. (Ed.). (1999). *The pilgrim's tale* (T. A. Smith, Trans.). New York: Paulist Press.

11. Oman, D. (2010). Similarity in diversity? Four shared functions of integrative contemplative practice systems. In T. G. Plante (Ed.), *Contemplative practices in action—spirituality, meditation, and health* (pp. 7–16). Oxford, England: Praeger.

12. Oman, D. (2013). Spiritual modeling and the social learning of spirituality and religion. In K. I. Pargament (Ed.), *APA handbook of psychology, religion and spirituality, Volume 1, Context, theory, and research* (pp. 187–204). Washington, DC: American Psychological Association.

13. Oman, D., & Thoresen, C. E. (2003). Spiritual modeling: A key to spiritual and religious growth? *International Journal for the Psychology of Religion, 13*(3), 149–165.

14. Oman, D., & Thoresen, C. E. (2007). How does one learn to be spiritual? The neglected role of spiritual modeling in health. In T. G. Plante & C. E. Thoresen (Eds.), *Spirit, science and health: How the spiritual mind fuels physical wellness* (pp. 39–54). Westport, CT: Praeger.

15. Plante, T. G. (2009). *Spiritual practices in psychotherapy: Thirteen tools for enhancing psychological health.* Washington, DC: American Psychological Association.

16. Bandura, A. (1986). *Social foundations of thoughts and action.* Englewood Cliffs, NJ: Prentice-Hall.

17. Bandura, A. (2003). On the psychosocial impact and mechanisms of spiritual modeling. *The International Journal for the Psychology of Religion, 13,* 167–173.

18. Oman, D., & Thoresen, C. E. (2003). Authors' response: "The many frontiers of spiritual modeling." *The International Journal for the Psychology of Religion, 13*(3), 197–213.

19. Oman, D., Thoresen, C. E., Park, C. L., Shaver, P. R., Hood, R. W., & Plante, T. G. (2009). How does one become spiritual? The spiritual modeling inventory of life environments (SMILE). *Mental Health, Religion and Culture, 12*(5), 427–456.

20. (Brémault-)Phillips, S. (2009). *Re-reading* The way of a pilgrim*: A research project utilizing contemplative psychology* (Doctoral thesis). Saint Paul University, Ottawa, ON.

21. (Brémault-)Phillips, S. (2009). Anonymous (mid-nineteenth century) *The way of a pilgrim.* In A. Holder (Ed.), *Christian spirituality: The classics* (pp. 293–304). New York: Routledge.

22. (Brémault-)Phillips, S. (2005). *The way of a pilgrim*: A synopsis of recent scholarship on a spiritual classic. *Logos: A Journal of Eastern Christian Studies, 46*(3–4), 525–542.

23. Palmer, G. E. H., Sherrard, P., & Ware, K. (Trans.). (1979–1995). *The philokalia: The complete text* (4 vols.). London, England: Faber & Faber.

CHAPTER NINE

Expressive Writing as a Spiritual Practice to Promote Resilience and Posttraumatic Growth among Disaster-Exposed Pregnant Women

*Suzette Brémault-Phillips, Ashley Pike,
Joanne K. Olson, and David M. Olson*

Pregnancy as a Sacred and Spiritual Time

Pregnancy and childbirth can be one of the most remarkable and enlightening events that a woman experiences.[1,2] Some suggest that nothing is more spiritually tied to our humanness than childbirth—the entrance of new life and taking of the first breath.[3-5] Moloney[6] contends that "cross-culturally and throughout history, pregnancy and childbirth have been perceived as spiritual events because of the miraculous processes involved" (p. 1), with pregnancy itself being an opportunity to contemplate the "nature of the experience and to deepen or renew spiritual connectedness" (p. 151).[7] In most cultures, pregnancy confers particular status to pregnant women[8] and is accompanied by customs often rooted in traditional medicine or religion. As with many of the wisdom traditions, pregnancy and childbirth are considered to be sacred from a Judeo-Christian perspective, and value is placed on the fundamental role of women in the giving of the sacred gift of new life.[9]

Childbearing and motherhood may offer the quintessential context in which to enhance one's spirituality. The spirituality of pregnancy and childbirth is related both to the "transcendence of a hope and dream into a real, living being"[10] and the profundity of connections cultivated with self, partner, child, family, and the sacred or transcendent. Spiritual activities engaged in during pregnancy can deepen a woman's spirituality and promote self-care.[11] Such activities often include making personal sacrifices for the greater good and well-being of an unborn child (e.g., dietary restrictions, abstinence from select activities). Women may also discuss spiritual matters with others, frequent places that enable them to feel closer to God or a higher power, meditate or pray, read spiritual material, practice forgiveness, and ascribe spiritual meaning to various experiences.[7] Journaling is a further practice that can help pregnant women connect with self and the sacred or transcendent. It is anticipated that once a woman has established connections with her spiritual self, she is more able to connect with her child before, during, and after the birth.[10] Establishing such connections may be all the more important if women are exposed to stressful events or disasters in the course of their pregnancy that can affect them and their unborn children.

Impacts of Disasters on Mother and Child

There is increasing awareness that life experiences, particularly negative ones, can affect maternal and child well-being, health, and pregnancy outcomes. While positive experiences can cultivate a sense of connection and well-being, stressful events such as natural disasters can be nothing shy of disruptive and traumatic. Wildfires, hurricanes, tropical storms, ice storms, earthquakes, and floods routinely affect populations, inclusive of pregnant women. Between 1980 and 2015, 11,538 natural disasters were reported (including Hurricane Katrina, the Haiti and Nepal earthquakes, the Japan tsunami, and the Philippines typhoon).[12] In the Americas alone, 2,762 natural disasters occurred between 1980 and 2015,[12] and six consecutive hurricanes formed in 2017.[13] Global natural disasters reported in 2016 included 315 events and caused insured losses of US$54 billion;[14] the disaster risk has been predicted to increase if global trends continue.[14] Damage, destruction, and human suffering caused by natural disasters can be tremendous, and the capacity of local communities to respond to basic needs,[15,16] let alone particular needs associated with pregnancy and childbirth, can be greatly compromised. As a result, natural disasters can leave pregnant women and their unborn children vulnerable.

The impact of large-scale disasters on the general population, and pregnant women more specifically, is staggering. Individuals may suffer losses of loved ones, health, possessions, homes, financial stability, social supports, and resources needed for daily living.[17,18] The psychological and spiritual imprinting and fallout that results can range from being minimal and short-lived to long term and psychopathological.[19] How a person deals with a disaster, and whether or not they bounces back or grows from the event, can be dependent on the person's coping abilities; perceptions; beliefs; choices; and relationships with self, others, the world, and the sacred or transcendent.[20-22] It is noteworthy that, among those who experience the same disaster, women tend to experience more acute symptoms of posttraumatic stress disorder (PTSD) than do men.[23,24] Pregnant women can be even more vulnerable to stress in light of their concern not only for themselves, their spouses, and possibly other children, but also for their unborn child.

Stress related to natural disasters during pregnancy can result in negative pregnancy outcomes, preterm births, childhood cognitive delays, and potential intergenerational implications.[25-30] Research conducted on pregnant women who experienced a flood in Poland found that 53.3 percent of participants experienced a miscarriage, fetal death, or other adverse outcomes in addition to stress-related physical and mental complications.[31] Badakhsh, Harville, and Banerjee,[32] who interviewed pregnant women living in New Orleans during Hurricane Katrina, heard that the hurricane destroyed normalcy, shattered expectations, created uncertainty within families and homes and around childbirth and childcare, raised concerns about living in New Orleans post Katrina, and left women trying to cope with establishing a new life while simultaneously bringing a new life into the world.

Spirituality: Similarities between Pregnancy and Exposure to Disasters

Interestingly, experiences of pregnancy and exposure to natural disasters share some things in common regarding spirituality. Well-being, perspectives, and function in both circumstances can be affected by a person's spiritual and religious worldviews (including beliefs, values, and understandings of the sacred or transcendent).[33-35] Questions of a spiritual or existential nature can arise in the course of events (e.g., "Where is love and God?"),[36] as can spiritual struggles (e.g., challenges to one's beliefs). Spiritual beliefs can be either strengthened or challenged in either circumstance, with some individuals relying on their beliefs to make meaning of and adjust to new realities.[37,38] Religious and spiritual practices, rituals, and processes may be engaged in to help people cope with, minimize negative impacts of, and recover from events.[17,39] Renewed connections with self, others, and the sacred or transcendent on a potentially deeper and more genuine level can result,[40] as can an increased altruistic reflex, in the course of events. Further, both pregnancy and exposure to natural disasters may be times when people experience pain, suffering, and loss of control. Finding themselves stripped of the familiar and material, and faced with significant lifestyle changes, they may be left with nothing more than hope and trust in what and who they can and cannot see. Pregnant women exposed to natural disasters often live these experiences more intensely. They can also be more spiritually attuned and readily draw on spiritual resources, practices, and communities as a means of coping and thriving.

Resilience—Bouncing Back and Growing from Life's Stresses

There has been growing interest in the ability of people and communities—including pregnant women—to be resilient and experience growth in the face of trauma.[41] Resilience is the capacity to flex without fracturing—"the process of adapting well in the face of adversity, trauma, tragedy, threats or significant sources of stress."[42] It involves reaching out to others and opportunities that support growth and finding and negotiating culturally meaningful resources that sustain well-being and recovery from trauma.[43] Posttraumatic growth (PTG) refers to positive, meaningful psychological changes that an individual experiences as a result of struggling with stressful and traumatic events.[44,45] It is associated with an increased sense of personal strength and self-awareness, an appreciation of life and other individuals, and spiritual growth.[46] Findings from studies of PTG among adults who have experienced trauma (e.g., former prisoners of war, survivors of assault, college students, war veterans, refugees, and individuals with medical conditions and injuries) suggest that more than 50 percent of survivors report PTG in one or more domains.[41] If appropriate resources can be tapped and interventions made available, this bodes well for pregnant women exposed to natural disasters.

Associations appear to exist between resilience, PTSD, and PTG.[41] As individuals who are resilient are less likely to experience posttraumatic stress and develop PTSD, there is a presumed negative causal link between resilience and PTSD.[47,48] This negative association also seems to exist between resilience and PTG, with highly resilient individuals tending to both rapidly recover and return to baseline functioning following trauma exposure and experience less PTG.[49] For PTG to occur, it is thought that a person may need to experience a significant threat to or shattering of their views about self, others, the world, and the sacred or transcendent such that deep existential questions arise.[50] New realizations about one's worldview, beliefs, and values stimulate growth and alter how one relates to self and others, makes choices, and engages in the world. As profound existential questioning may not arise in the course of traumatic events for people who are more resilient, PTG may be more modest.

Spirituality, Resilience, and Posttraumatic Growth

According to Tsai and colleagues,[41] spirituality and religion have consistently been found to be related to PTG in adults and children[51,52] (although, subsequent to trauma, negative religious coping and practices can be employed or negative religious beliefs develop[51,53] that may hinder recovery and growth). Some people who experience trauma develop greater existential awareness[54] that enhances their personal, religious, or spiritual beliefs. Others seek spiritual models that provide examples of how to face and overcome challenging or traumatic circumstances. Spiritual or religious practices and rituals may also cultivate a sense of awareness of, connection to, and relationship with self, others, and the sacred and/or transcendent. Journaling is one such practice that can help build resilience, cultivate PTG, and enable people to overcome PTSD. As a result, it may be beneficial for pregnant women in general, and those exposed to natural disasters more particularly, to engage in the practice of expressive writing.

The Practice of Expressive Writing—Its Relation to Trauma and Resilience

Recent research into the serious and long-term effects of trauma has led to efforts to identify brief and accessible interventions to support those who experience trauma and enhance resilience. Since the 1980s, James W. Pennebaker has tested and refined a simple expressive writing intervention to help people deal with stressors.[55,56] Short bursts of writing (i.e., 15–20 minutes) appear to be sufficient to allow for emotional disclosure (the active ingredient in the intervention)[57–59] and improve biochemical markers of physical and immune functioning.[60,61] A self-reflective learning activity, expressive writing accesses innermost thoughts and feelings and allows for review and cognitive processing of what has been written. In so doing, it relieves anxiety and weakens the relationship between intrusive thoughts and distress.[62] Worries are offloaded from working memory, and distracting effects on cognition are relieved.[63] Expressive writing has also been found to cultivate both resilience (with people with the greatest resilience tending to make the most meaning from their experiences[64–66]) and optimism (viewing difficult times as temporary and as they are but not worse than they are). Further, it helps people identify what is most important in life and protects against depression.[67–70] The more individuals disclose about a traumatic experience, the better their likelihood of long-term health.[71] Expressive writing is being encouraged as a means for such disclosure.

Writing and journaling are considered by many to be spiritual practices.[72–74] Found in neostoic writings and early Judeo-Christian pastoral and spiritual direction literature,[75] this reflective and contemplative practice involves setting aside time to center the self and focus attention.[76] While engaging in the practice, the person can reconnect with self, others, and the sacred and/or transcendent as well as examine thoughts, feelings, and conscience.[75] Life reviews and meaning making of life events can also occur. Resilience, spirituality, and performance have been found to be fostered by writing and journaling.[74]

Case Study: Fort McMurray, Alberta, Wildfires

Recently, researchers at the University of Alberta, University of Lethbridge, and McGill University implemented an online expressive writing intervention with women who were pregnant at the time of, or soon to conceive following, the May 2016 wildfire in Fort McMurray–Wood Buffalo (FMWB), Alberta. The wildfires that hit the oil-sand-producing region of Alberta charred more than 1.43 million acres of land, destroyed approximately 10 percent of Fort McMurray (including more than 2,400 homes and other structures), generated economic losses of US$4.5 billion and insured losses of US$2.8 billion, and prompted the largest evacuation in the history of Alberta. Among the 88,000 residents forced to evacuate FMWB were an estimated 1,250 women who were pregnant and 600 who were likely to conceive in the following six months. Of the pregnant women, some gave birth under extreme conditions during the evacuation; others had preterm births or delivered in unplanned circumstances. The wildfire's devastating impact ensured that it was the costliest natural disaster in Canadian history.[14]

Signs of stress appeared immediately following the wildfire in some individuals and manifested weeks and months later for others. In actuality, it may be years before the full impact of the event is apparent. Preliminary results from the study indicate that more than 70 percent of the pregnant and postpartum study participants experience posttraumatic stress, and 30 percent exhibit symptoms consistent with a diagnosis of PTSD. This rate is two to three times higher than for women in other natural disasters (2008 Iowa, United States, floods; 2001 Queensland, Australia, floods; January 1998 Quebec, Canada, ice storm) and is associated with adverse outcomes. Overall, the disaster has tested people's resilience and ability to cope while also being an opportunity for PTG.

A key objective of the study was to determine the impact of expressive writing on the perceived stress and resilience of pregnant women exposed to the natural disaster. After completing a battery of questionnaires and being randomly assigned to one of three groups (writing, expressive writing, and no writing), recruited participants in both of the writing groups wrote online for 15–20 minutes on four consecutive days, prompted with specific guiding questions. The research questions informing data collection and analysis included (1) What thoughts, feelings, themes, experiences, actions, relationships, and factors did the pregnant women write about that reflect aspects of resilience? and (2) In their postjournaling reflections, how effective did the women find journaling to be? Responses on the preintervention question-naires and journal entries were qualitatively analyzed.

Preliminary Findings

Preliminary findings suggest that expressive writing was helpful for preg-nant women facing traumatic stress. A majority of the women found that the practice provided an opportunity to reflect on, connect with, and better understand themselves. Women wrote of the mental, physical, emotional, and relational toll of unresolved issues associated with experiences related and unrelated to the wildfire, together with their coping strategies. The pro-cess of writing helped them to externalize thoughts and feelings (including of things they had not previously shared), reevaluate their responses to life experiences, and bring closure to past events. For many, it enabled them to consider what was most important to them and stimulated personal growth. Writing also served as a catalyst for seeking support. While they indicated that it was difficult to find time to write and to connect with their thoughts and feelings, the majority of respondents were grateful for having done so; only a minority appeared neutral in their appraisal.

Several broad themes emerged in the women's writing, including resil-ience, expressive writing as a practice, emotional connectedness, connection to self, posttraumatic growth, social connection, and spiritual connection and eagerness. Following is a synopsis of responses elicited by questions asked of study participants.

Resilience

The majority of women clearly appreciated the need to be resilient in the face of the natural disaster. Many were also aware of the potential impact of stress and trauma on their unborn child and made conscious efforts to remain as calm as possible. The importance of social connection and relating to other community members who shared their experience was evident; con-necting enabled them to remain strong and grounded amid uncertain cir-cumstances. Engagement in spiritual practices (e.g., self-reflection through expressive writing, speaking with others, being grateful, employing breath-ing techniques, shifting focus to the positive, meditating, praying, reading, yoga, and therapy) also helped them cope with the stress.

The Practice of Expressive Writing

Expressive writing was clearly an effective spiritual practice. As an inter-vention, writing versus no writing was found to be associated with positive outcomes on all measures of stress and depression. PTSD, stress, and depression scores improved regardless of whether one was in the writing group (writing about lifestyle and diet) or the expressive writing group (writing about the fire, past trauma, and conflict). Positive effects of writing on maternal mood were still evident at four months after baseline data collection and completion of the four-day writing intervention. Many women reported that writing enabled them to self-reflect. One participant wrote, "To help me, I wrote. I felt the pages of my diary would really hear me out." Another participant reported the sense of relief she felt from writing about things she had not previously shared with anyone: "It was a good opportunity for me to reflect on situations at hand and get a bit of closure. It also helped me reevaluate how I responded to some things in my daily life and in the past." The women indicated that writing definitely helped them to "grow as a person."

Emotional Connectedness

The women openly shared their emotions and how they were dealing with them. Emotions ranged from anger, anxiety, frustration, sadness, guilt, and vulnerability, to relief, gratitude, love, appreciation, optimism, contentment, and happiness. Many of the women wrote of feeling stronger emotional connections to their spouses/partners following the fire as well as a desire to spend time with their children. Some of the women also commented on support received from parents and emotional connections with those who also lived through the experience of the fire and evacuation.

The importance of regulating emotions, practicing patience, and managing negativity was evident in the participants' writings. They felt that avoiding comparisons and maintaining a realistic perspective and composure for the sake of the unborn baby was a priority. Many self-regulated by practicing deep breathing and positive self-talk, managing fear and negativity, remaining calm, and accepting that some circumstances are beyond their control.

While many of the women acknowledged that their resilience enabled them to cope, others did not. Some women reported that they had yet to discuss the impact of the fire and evacuation: "I don't discuss how intensely it has affected me with anyone." "I don't think I have 100% dealt with it. I just try to put it out of my mind. The fact that I haven't dealt with it will catch up with me eventually I know. I would probably benefit from speaking to someone." These revelations demonstrate the need for intentional and timely interventions after trauma.

Connection to Self

Writing enabled the women to connect with themselves. They described a newfound sense of agency and belief in their capacity. They also wrote of intentionally focusing on themselves, asking for help, making decisions, managing their stress levels, and changing their thought processes. While they quickly came to realize and accept that they were not in control of their reality, they also grew in independence and self-confidence. The women reported realizing their own self-worth, which helped them remain grounded in themselves and their values. The experience caused them to reevaluate their meaning and purpose in life. A sense of vision, clarity regarding future goals, and personal values resulted. These realizations enabled them to be more conscious of their priorities and intentional regarding choices and actions that aligned with their goals. Further, most women came to a new appreciation for everything they had, with one woman stating, "During that time, I was . . . able to let go of my material goods," as relationships clearly became the priority. Many also had a change in mind-set, shifted their focus to the positive, and avoided negative people and situations. Participants reported, "I try to fill each day with happier thoughts!," "To cope, I focused on the positive. I tried very hard not to stress," "I like to be realistic about things," and "I told myself I was going to be okay." Further, the women commented on their deepened sense of gratitude, optimism, and happiness: "Gratitude has been a gigantic source of happiness and healing for me and I try to implement it daily in my life. I've had many conflicts and problems in my young life, but I feel this one stands out amongst others mainly because it was a turning point in my life that led me to a healthier me—mind, body and spirit." Another woman shared, "During that time, I was most thankful to simply be alive (I didn't think we were going to be able to leave the hospital as the fire got closer and closer)."

Posttraumatic Growth

The women wrote about learning new strategies for dealing with negative situations and stress and making healthy lifestyle changes. Their writings reflected an increased ability to reason, problem solve, and be resourceful and ready for change. They wrote about fact finding, searching for realistic options, making smart decisions, and solving or eliminating problems as they arose. Many utilized appropriate resources and mobilized and took action, including evacuating early to get ahead of traffic and minimize stress. Others began planning for a potential future evacuation while reassuring themselves of the low likelihood of such a recurrence. Some were emboldened to remove themselves from negative situations and speak with those on the other side of conflicts. They also exhibited strengths-based aptitudes. The women drew on inner strength and were persistent in resolving conflict. Their determination to heal, improve relationships, or work toward a goal was clear in their writing. Adaptability was evident in their finding of a "new normal" following the fire, adjusting to new or changed jobs and situations, and receiving constructive criticism and growing from it. Healthy lifestyle changes were also stimulated by the event, with many women choosing to focus on health during the evacuation by drinking water, eating healthy food, breathing, meditating, and exercising. One woman reported, "What's helped me the most is doing healthy things for me." Some reported that they were motivated to do so by their unborn child.

Social Connection

Social connectedness was frequently addressed in the women's expressive writing. The women noted that the evacuation resulted in the formation of new friendships and deepening of existing ones with partners, family, and friends. Many found strength, support, and enriched connections with their husbands. They also bonded over the shared experience with family, friends, community members, and coworkers. To cope with the fire, evacuation, and displacement, women ensured that they created quality family time, initiated conversations, and disclosed emotions and thoughts to loved ones. One woman stated, "Staying in touch more frequently with my parents has helped me." Another woman wrote, "Many of my personal relationships changed after the fire. I already knew some members of my community, but after the fire our relationships became stronger. I made really good friends and that is definitely a positive outcome."

Women wrote of the beauty of and necessity for collaboration as a result of the wildfire, describing the level of community spirit felt during this time as "incredible." Residents of FMWB selflessly came together to support one another (e.g., picking up neighbors from communities that were ablaze, opening up their homes to evacuees, helping one another prepare their residences for reentry, and jointly rebuilding the community).

Spiritual Connection and Eagerness

In addition to the aforementioned ways in which expressive writing helped women connect, cultivate resilience, and grow, it also helped them gain a deepened sense of spiritual connection and eagerness. In their writings, women noted exploring and connecting with their spirituality and reevaluating what gives them a sense of meaning and purpose. Many participants indicated that they found strength in prayer and faith: "I would pray and have found that my faith gives me lots of strength." "Praying and my relationship with God has gotten deeper." Numerous women related that they prayed (some for the first time); practiced meditation, yoga, and conscious breathing; read spiritual books; and found strength in their spiritual tradition and community during the evacuation and reentry.

Potential Areas of Impact

As we write this chapter, there have been recent hurricanes and floods in Texas, Florida, and Puerto Rico, and fires in the wine country of California. There seems to be no end to disasters and ensuing devastation to people's property and lives. While everyone in these disasters suffers immensely, we are especially aware of the many children and pregnant women in these populations.

This chapter has contributed to the literature by focusing on the resilience and personal growth of pregnant women exposed to natural disasters. Preliminary findings have helped us to better understand the impact of trauma on pregnant women and ways in which the spiritual practice of expressive writing can support self-awareness, well-being, resilience, and PTG. As a simple intervention, this practice could be encouraged during pregnancy and childbirth to support pregnant women as well as during and following natural disasters as a cost-effective and easily administered intervention to help people both manage stress and grow from potentially catastrophic experiences.

The expressive writing intervention provided study participants with a safe, anonymous outlet to convey their thoughts and emotions regarding the experience of the fire and evacuation as well as their life in general. Many women found the exercise to be effective, helping them to connect with experiences and feelings they may have detached from. Emotional disclosure through expressive writing enabled them to experience social, relational, and health benefits. It also invited reflection on the importance of relationships, resilience practices and strategies, adaptability, composure, emotional connectedness, and spiritual practices in general. PTG was evident in descriptions by the women regarding how the experience of the fire gave them a new perspective on life and a greater appreciation of belongings and relationships with self, others, and the transcendent. Others described growth and collaboration within the community as well as psychosocial and spiritual strategies for coping with negative situations.

Implications

Much can be done to reduce the vulnerability of populations living in areas where natural disasters occur.[75] Future risks can be prevented, existing risks reduced, and the resilience of communities fostered. Research has highlighted the need to build resilience within communities as a means of preparing them in advance for potential natural disasters and as a counterbalance to social and individual vulnerabilities. This includes pregnant women and children exposed to natural disasters who are among society's most vulnerable. Agencies have become increasingly compelled to consider how to cultivate resiliency.[19]

While exposure to natural disasters undoubtedly affects pregnant women and their children, interventions prior to, during, and following a traumatic event may well support their ability to bounce back and grow from life events. There is evidence to suggest that spiritual and religious practices, such as expressive writing, can be supportive both during the sacred time of pregnancy and childbearing as well as during natural disasters. Pregnant women exposed to disasters may benefit from engagement in spiritual practices. Based on the research discussed in this chapter, we recommend that expressive writing be used in routine prenatal and perinatal care as well as being a standard intervention before and after disaster to mitigate posttraumatic stress symptoms and foster resilience and posttraumatic growth. Such practices may help women connect to self, others, and the sacred or transcendent and adjust to changing life circumstances, whatever the cause. In the words of C. S. Lewis, "When we lose one blessing, another is often most unexpectedly given in its place."[77] Expressive writing may be a way to recognize and process extraordinary blessings amid variable and potentially traumatic life circumstances.

References

1. Etowa, J. B. (2012). Becoming a mother: The meaning of childbirth for African-Canadian woman. *Contemporary Nurse, 41*(1), 28–40.

2. Uguz, F., Gezginc, K., Zeytinci, I. E., Karatayli, S., Askin, R., Guler, O., & Gecici, O. (2007). Obsessive-compulsive disorder in pregnant women during the third trimester of pregnancy. *Comprehensive Psychiatry, 48*(1), 441–445.

3. Ayers-Gould, J. N. (2000). Spirituality in birth: Creating sacred space within the medical model. *International Journal of Childbirth Education, 15,* 14–17.

4. Baumiller, R. C. (2002). Spiritual development during a first pregnancy. *International Journal of Childbirth Education, 17,* 7.

5. Golberg, B. (1998). Connection: An exploration of spirituality in nursing care. *Journal of Advanced Nursing, 27,* 836–842.

6. Moloney, S. (2007). Dancing with the wind: A methodological approach to researching women's spirituality around menstruation and birth. *International Journal of Qualitative Methods, 6*(1), Article 7.

7. Jesse, D. E., Schoneboom, C., & Blanchard, A. (2007). The effect of faith and spirituality on pregnancy: A content analysis. *Journal of Holistic Nursing, 25,* 151–158.

8. Womack, M. (2010). *The anthropology of health and healing.* Plymouth, England: AltaMira Press.

9. Balin, J. (1988). The sacred dimensions of pregnancy and birth. *Qualitative Sociology, 11*(4), 275–301.

10. Ayers-Gould, J. (2000). Spirituality in birth: Creating sacred space within the medical model. *International Journal of Childbirth Education, 15*(1), 14–17.

11. Callister, L. C., & Khalaf, I. (2010). Spirituality in childbearing women. *The Journal of Perinatal Education, 19*(2), 16–24.

12. Center for Research on the Epidemiology of Disasters (CRED). (2017). *EM-DAT: The International Disaster Database.* Université catholique de Louvain Brussels, Belgium. Retrieved on March 12, 2018, from www.emdat.be

13. United Nations International Strategy for Disaster Reduction (UNISDR). (2015). *The Pocket GAR 2015.* Retrieved from http://www.preventionweb.net /englilsh/hyogo/gar/2015/en/home/GAR_pocket/Pocket%20GAR_3.html (link no longer active)

14. Aon. (2016). *Annual global climate and catastrophe report.* Retrieved on March 12, 2018, from http://thoughtleadership.aonbenfield.com/Documents /20170117-ab-if-annual-climate-catastrophe-report.pdf

15. Varghese, S. B. (2010). Cultural, ethical, and spiritual implications of natural disasters from the survivors' perspective. *Critical Care Nursing Clinics of North America, 22*(4), 515–522.

16. Ronan, K. R., & Johnston, D. M. (2005). *Promoting community resilience in disasters: The role of schools, youths, and families.* New York: Springer.

17. Norris, F. H., Friedman, M. J., Watson, P. J., Byrne, C. M., Diaz, E., & Kaniasty, K. (2002). 60,000 disaster victims speak: Part 1. An empirical review of the empirical literature, 1981–2001. *Psychiatry, 65*(3), 207–239.

18. Aten, J. D., O'Grady, K. A., Milstein, G., Boan, D., & Schruba, A. (2014). Spiritually oriented disaster psychology. *Spirituality in Clinical Practice, 1*(1), 20.

19. Abramson, D. M., Grattan, L. M., Mayer, B., Colten, C. E., Arosema, F. A., Bedimo-Rung, A., & Lichtveld, M. (2015). The resilience activation framework: A conceptual model of how access to social resources promotes adaptation and rapid recovery in post-disaster settings. *The Journal of Behavioral Health Services & Research, 42*(1), 42–57.

20. Kalayjian, A., Kanazi, R. L., Aberson, C. L., & Feygin, L. (2002). A cross-cultural study of the psychosocial and spiritual impact of natural disaster. *International Journal of Group Tensions, 31*(2), 175–186.

21. Roberts, A. R. (Ed.). (2005). *Crisis intervention handbook: Assessment, treatment, and research* (3rd ed.). New York: Oxford University Press.

22. Calhoun, L. G., & Tedeschi, R. G. (2006). The foundations of post-traumatic growth: An expanded framework. In L. G. Calhoun & R. G. Tedeschi (Eds.), *Handbook of posttraumatic growth: Research and practice* (pp. 1–23). Mahwah, NJ: Penguin.

23. Verger, P., Rotily, M., Hunault, C., Brenot, J., Baruffol, E., & Bard, D. (2003). Assessment of exposure to a flood disaster in a mental-health study. *Journal of Exposure Analysis and Environmental Epidemiology, 13*, 436–442.

24. Galea, S., Brewin, C. R., Gruber, M., Jones, R., King, L. A., & Kessler, R. C. (2007). Exposure to hurricane-related stressors and mental illness after Hurricane Katrina. *Archives of General Psychology, 64*, 1427–1434.

25. Glover, V. (2011). Annual research review: Prenatal stress and the origins of psychopathology: An evolutionary perspective. *Journal of Child Psychology and Psychiatry, 52*(4), 356–367.

26. Graignic-Philippe, R., Dayan, J., Chokron, S., Jacquet, A. Y., & Tordjman, S. (2014). Effects of prenatal stress on fetal and child development: A critical literature review. *Neuroscience and Biobehavioral Review, 43,* 137–162.

27. Talge, N. M., Neal, C., & Glover, V. (2007). Antenatal maternal stress and long-term effects on child neurodevelopment: How and why? *Journal of Child Psychology and Psychiatry, 48,* 245–261.

28. Christiaens, I., Hegadoren, K., & Olson, D. M. (2015). Adverse childhood experiences are associated with spontaneous preterm birth: A case-control study. *BMC Medicine, 13,* 124.

29. Brock, R. L., O'Hara, M. W., Hart, K. J., McCabe, J. E., Williamson, J. A., Laplante, D. P., . . . King, S. (2014). Partner support and maternal depression in the context of the Iowa Floods. *Journal of Family Psychology, 28*(6), 832–843.

30. Dancause, K. N., Laplante, D. P., Oremus, C., Fraser, S., Brunet, A., & King, S. (2011). Disaster-related prenatal maternal stress influences birth outcomes: Project Ice Storm. *Early Human Development, 87*(12), 813–820.

31. Neuberg, M., Pawlosek, W., Lopuszanski, M., & Neuberg, J. (1998). The analysis of the course of pregnancy, delivery and postpartum women touched by flood disaster in Kotlin Klodzki in July 1997. *Ginekologia Polska, 69,* 866–870.

32. Badakhsh, R., Harville, E., & Banerjee, B. (2010). The childbearing experience during a natural disaster. *Journal of Obstetric, Gynecologic, & Neonatal Nursing, 39,* 489–497.

33. Pargament, K. I. (2011). *Spiritually integrated psychotherapy—Understanding and addressing the sacred.* New York: Guilford Press.

34. Moriarty, G. L., & Davis, E. B. (2012). Client God images: Theory, research, and clinical practice. In J. Aten, K. O'Grady, & E. Worthington, Jr. (Eds.), *The psychology of religion and spirituality for clinicians: Using research in your practice* (pp. 131–160). New York: Routledge.

35. O'Grady, K. A., & Richards, P. S. (2008). God image and theistic psychotherapy. *Journal of Spirituality and Mental Health, 9,* 183–209. doi:10.1300 /J515v09n03_09

36. Koenig H. G. (2006). *In the wake of disaster: Religious responses to terrorism and catastrophe.* Philadelphia, PA: Templeton Press.

37. Peterson, C., & Seligman, M. E. P. (2003). Character strengths before and after September 11. *Psychological Science, 14,* 381–384.

38. Aten, J. D., Moore, M., Denny, R. M., Bayne, T., Stagg, A., Owens, S., . . . Jones, C. (2008). God images following Hurricane Katrina in South Mississippi: An exploration study. *Journal of Psychological Theology.* Retrieved on March 12, 2018, from http://www.thefreelibrary.com/

39. Smith, B., Pargament, K., Brant, C., & Oliver, J. (2000). Noah revisited: Religious coping by church members and the impact of the 1993 Midwest flood. *Journal of Community Psychology, 28,* 169–186.

40. Rigler, S. Y. (2005). After disaster. Aish.com. Retrieved on March 12, 2018, from http://www.aish.com/ci/be/48892392.html doi:10.1002/(SICI)1520 -6629(200003)28:23.0.CO;2-I

41. Tsai, J., Harpaz-Rotem, I., Pietrzak, R. H., & Southwick, S. M. (2017). Trauma resiliency and posttraumatic growth. In S. N. Gold (Ed.), *APA handbook of trauma psychology: Trauma practice* (pp. 89–113). Washington, DC: American Psychological Association.

42. American Psychological Association. (n.d.). The road to resilience. Retrieved on March 12, 2018, from http://www.apa.org/helpcenter/road-resilience .aspx

43. Fergus, S., & Zimmerman, M. A. (2005). Adolescent resilience: A framework for understanding healthy development in the face of risk. *Annual Review of Public Health, 26,* 399–419.

44. Zoellner, T., & Maercker, A. (2006). Posttraumatic growth in clinical psychology—a critical review and introduction of a two component model. *Clinical Psychology Review, 26,* 626–653. http://dx.doi.org/ 10.1016/j.cpr.2006.01.008

45. Tedeschi, R. G., & McNally, R. J. (2011). Can we facilitate posttraumatic growth in combat veterans? *American Psychologist, 66*(1), 19.

46. Tedeschi, R. G., Park, C. L., & Calhoun, L. G. (Eds.). (1998). *Posttraumatic growth: Positive changes in the aftermath of crisis.* Mahwah, NJ: Lawrence Erlbaum Associates.

47. Paton, D., Violanti, J. M., & Smith, L. M. (2003). *Promoting capabilities to manage posttraumatic stress: Perspectives on resilience.* Springfield, IL: Charles C. Thomas Publisher.

48. Rutter, M. (1985). Resilience in the face of adversity. Protective factors and resistance to psychiatric disorder. *The British Journal of Psychiatry, 147*(6), 598–611.

49. Levine, S. Z., Laufer, A., Stein, E., Hamama-Raz, Y., & Solomon, Z. (2009). Examining the relationship between resilience and posttraumatic growth. *Journal of Traumatic Stress, 22,* 282–286. http://dx.doi.org/ 10.1002/jts.20409

50. Tedeschi, R. G., & Kilmer, R. P. (2005). Assessing strengths, resilience, and growth to guide clinical interventions. *Professional Psychology: Research and Practice, 36,* 230–237.

51. Shaw, A., Joseph, S., & Linley, P. A. (2005). Religion, spirituality, and posttraumatic growth: A systematic review. *Mental Health, Religion, and Culture, 8,* 1–11. http://dx.doi.org/10.1080/1367467032000157981

52. Tsai, J., El-Gabalawy, R., Sledge, W. H., Southwick, S. M., & Pietrzak, R. H. (2015). Post-traumatic growth among veterans in the USA: Results from the National Health and Resilience in Veterans Study. *Psychological Medicine, 45,* 165–179. http://dx.doi.org/10.1017/S0033291714001202

53. Pargament, K. I., Smith, B. W., Koenig, H. G., & Perez, L. (1998). Patterns of positive and negative religious coping with major life stressors. *Journal for the Scientific Study of Religion, 37,* 710–724. http://dx.doi.org /10.2307/1388152

54. Yalom, I. D., & Lieberman, M. A. (1991). Bereavement and heightened existential awareness. *Psychiatry: Interpersonal and Biological Processes, 54,* 334–345.

55. Pennebaker, J. W. (2007). *Emotion, disclosure and health* (5th ed.). Washington, DC: American Psychological Services.

56. Pennebaker, J. W., Chung C. K., Ireland, M. E., Gonzales, N. A., & Booth, R. J. (2007). *The LIWC 2007 Manual*. Austin, TX: LIWC.

57. Lange, A., Rietdijk, D., Hudcovicova, M., van de Ven. J.-P., Schrieken, B., & Emmelkamp, P. M. G. (2003). Interapy: A controlled randomized trial of the standardized treatment of posttraumatic stress through the internet. *Journal of Consulting and Clinical Psychology, 71*(5), 901–909.

58. Adams, K. (1996). Journal writing as a powerful adjunct to therapy. *Journal of Poetry Therapy, 10*(1), 31–37.

59. Adams, K. (1999). Writing as therapy. *Counseling and Human Development, 31*(5), 1–16.

60. Petrie, K. J., Booth, R. J., Pennebaker, J. W., Davison, K. P., & Thomas, M. G. (1995). Disclosure of trauma and immune response to a hepatitis B vaccination program. *Journal of Consulting Clinical Psychology, 63*(5), 787–792.

61. Baddeley, J. L., & Pennebaker, J. W. (2011). A postdeployment expressive writing intervention for military couples: A randomized controlled trial. *Journal of Trauma and Stress, 24*(5), 581–585.

62. Lepore, S. J. (1997). Expressive writing moderates the relation between intrusive thoughts and depressive symptoms. *Journal of Personality and Social Psychology, 73,* 1030–1037.

63. Schroder, H. S., Moran, T. P., & Moser, J. S. (2017). The effect of expressive writing on the error-related negativity among individuals with chronic worry. *Psychophysiology, 55*(2), 1–11. doi:10.1111/psyp.12990

64. Masten, A. S., & Coatsworth, J. D. (1998). The development of competence in favorable and unfavorable environments: Lessons from research on successful children. *American Psychologist, 53*(2), 205–220.

65. Borge, A. I., Motti-Stefanidi, F., & Masten, A. S. (2016). Resilience in developing systems: The promise of integrated approaches for understanding and facilitating positive adaptation to adversity in individuals and their families. *European Journal of Developmental Psychology, 13*(3), 293–296.

66. Masten, A. S. (2011). Resilience in children threatened by extreme adversity: Frameworks for research, practice, and translational synergy. *Development and Psychopathology, 23,* 493–506.

67. Mininni, D. (2005). *The emotional toolkit: 7 power-skills to nail your bad feelings.* New York: St. Martin's Press.

68. Reivich K., Gillham J. E., Chaplin, T. M., & Seligman, M. E. P. (2013). From helplessness to optimism: The role of resilience in treating and preventing depression in youth. In S. Goldstein & R. B. Brooks (Eds.), *Handbook of resilience in children* (pp. 201–214). New York: Springer.

69. Reivich, K., & Shatté, A. (2002). *The resilience factor: 7 essential skills for overcoming life's inevitable obstacles.* New York: Broadway Books.

70. Seligman, M. E. P., Reivich, K., Jaycox, L., & Gillham, J. (1995). *The optimistic child*. New York: Harper Perennial.

71. Pennebaker, J. W., Barger, S. D., & Tiebout, J. (1989). Disclosure of traumas and health among Holocaust survivors. *Psychosomatic Medicine, 51*(5), 577–589.

72. Cepero, H. (2015). *Journaling as a spiritual practice: Encountering God through attentive writing*. Westmont, IL: InterVarsity Press.

73. Hering, K. (2013). *Writing to wake the soul: Opening the sacred conversation within*. New York: Atria Books.

74. Reave, L. (2005). Spiritual values and practices related to leadership effectiveness. *The Leadership Quarterly, 16*(5), 655–687.

75. Global Facility for Disaster Reduction and Recovery (GFDRR). (2014). *Understanding risk in an evolving world: Emerging best practices in natural disaster risk assessment*. Retrieved on March 12, 2018, from http://www.preventionweb.net/publications/view/38130

76. Plante, T. G., Raz, A., & Oman, D. (2010). Introduction: Contemplative practices in action. In T. G. Plante (Ed.), *Contemplative practices in action—spirituality, meditation, and health*. Oxford, England: Praeger.

77. Lewis, C. S. (2008). *Yours, Jack: Spiritual direction from CS Lewis*. Grand Rapids, MI: Zondervan.

CHAPTER TEN

Mindfulness-Based Parenting Programs: Significance for Young Children Experiencing Adversity and Trauma

Barbara M. Burns

[The] challenge of mindful parenting is to find ways to nourish our children and ourselves, to remain true to the quest, the hero's journey that is a human life lived in awareness, across our entire life span, and so to grow into who we all are and can become for each other, for ourselves, and for the world.

—Kabat-Zinn and Kabat-Zinn[1]

For centuries, mindful practices have been a healing component in spiritual and religious traditions. Recent discoveries from the neurobiology of stress, children's resilience, and clinical psychology suggest that integrating spiritual practices of mindfulness and compassion into parenting programs may have a unique ability to strengthen parents' capacities for more nurturing parenting practices and promote resilience in children. This chapter describes recent advances in the theory and practice of mindfulness-based parenting programs (MBPP) and examines the potential of MBPPs to promote resilience and address some of the unique barriers to emotional well-being and mental health in culturally diverse families facing adversity and trauma.

Adversity, Trauma, and Resilience in Young Children

The adverse childhood experiences (ACEs) study by Felitti and colleagues explored the origins of risk factors that negatively affect adult physical and mental health.[2] Findings from this collaboration of Kaiser-Permanente and the Centers for Disease Control and Prevention have been widely recognized as some of the most important public health discoveries of the 21st century.[3,4] Felitti and colleagues examined adult health outcomes in relation to adverse childhood experiences in family life, such as domestic violence, substance abuse in the home, divorce, loss of parent (death or incarceration), abuse, neglect, family mental health problems, and racial/ethnic social rejection. They found that exposure to these ACEs was very common and linked to an array of social, emotional, and behavioral problems and long-term negative developmental outcomes. Felitti and colleagues analyses revealed that early childhood adversities show a dose-response relationship to mental and physical health outcomes.[2] The more ACEs experienced in early childhood, the more health and behavior problems in adulthood. The ACEs study confirmed what pediatricians and child-welfare professionals long suspected about the relation between early adversity and children's overall well-being and has led to a renewed interest in the study of adversity, trauma, and resilience across the life span.[3-6]

Recent discoveries from developmental neurobiology suggest that chronic stress from continued exposure to adversity and trauma in early childhood underlies many of the ACEs challenges to health and well-being.[4,5] Chronic stress in early childhood has been linked to deficits in children's brain architecture, disrupted brain response systems to fear and stress, and an array of social, emotional, cognitive, and behavioral delays.[3-6] In the United States, identified social, emotional, and behavioral problems in preschoolers have been estimated at 7 to 10 percent and include disorders in self-regulation, disruptive behavior, anxiety and mood, attention-deficit/hyperactivity disorders, and attachment.[3,4]

Although it has been well established that adversity and trauma in early childhood increase the frequency and severity of negative health outcomes, researchers have found variation in how individual children respond to cumulative risks.[6,7] Some children who face high levels of adversity exhibit positive trajectories in cognitive, emotional, and health outcomes.[6,7] These children are described in the research literature as demonstrating "resilience," as they show adaptability to stress and adversity. In childhood, they are able to manage and regulate emotions, deal with conflict, establish secure attachments, and show successful trajectories in school achievement.[6,7]

Ann Masten, a pioneer in the science of children's resilience, refers to this phenomenon of children showing resilience in the context of multiple, chronic, and interacting risks as the "ordinary magic of positive development."[7] Masten and her colleagues have led an extensive scientific effort to better understand the mechanisms of resilience and to identify individual, family, and community strengths that act as buffers to adversity and trauma and underlie children's trajectories of resilience. Masten has shown that resiliency is best viewed not as a personal trait but rather as a system of human competencies that allows for adaptation in the face of adversity. Masten's programmatic research has documented a complex set of risk and protective factors for healthy child and adolescent development. The findings from her work have provided a blueprint for interventionists working to identify and strengthen the competencies that underlie children's trajectories of resilience.[6–9]

Roots of Resilience

[Beginning at birth,] infants and their parents coregulate their social interactions by responding moment-to-moment to each other's affective and behavioral displays.

—Beeghly and Tronick[9]

To understand the roots of resilience, the early competencies that underlie the infant's ability to effectively manage stress and adversity, as well as how these competencies are strengthened in the context of the parent–infant relationship, must be considered within a developmental psychobiological framework.[6,8–9] The infant's brain-regulation system to manage stress is highly immature and highly malleable. Infants have an acute response to discomfort and do not have the neurobiological capacity to calm themselves. When parents consistently respond to their infant's stress, fear, and discomfort with sensitive care, they provide their infant with parent–infant mutual coregulation, a type of social scaffolding, which contributes to the neurobiological strategies that manage stress. This moment-to-moment coregulation also supports the infant's emerging ability to reset brain-regulation patterns following stress, fear, and discomfort. The infant's stress-regulation system, including foundational self-regulation and self-soothing skills, are actively shaped by the process of parent–infant mutual coregulation.[3,4,8,9]

However, the path from parent–infant mutual coregulation to a mature stress-regulation system is not simple and is affected by a wide array of risk and protective factors. According to infancy researchers, more than 70 percent of parent–infant interactions can best be characterized as *mismatches* in parent–infant mutual coregulation that cause varying levels of dysregulation and stress in the infant. Thus, the neurobiological strategies for managing stress, fear, and discomfort are learned primarily through the repair, or remediation, of *mismatches*. Mismatches in coregulation, when followed by repair, provide the infant with opportunities to learn to transition from a state of stress, fear, and discomfort to a state of comfort and well-being. Mature brain-regulation strategies to manage stress become established based on this frequently repeated process of the infant experiencing stress and dysregulation, parental repair, and a return to feelings of comfort and well-being.[3,4,6,8,9]

Added challenges to the path from parent–infant mutual coregulation to the infant's acquisition of a mature stress-regulation system come from the many genetic, biological, and environmental factors that affect the infant's regulatory system and ability to reset the system and transition from stress, fear, and discomfort to comfort and well-being.[3,4,6,10] Genetic and biological factors include the infant's ability to manage physiological states, the maturation of the infant's communication system, and many others. One of the most influential environmental factors affecting this path from coregulation to infant self-regulation is the parent's ability to recognize the infant's communication accurately and respond with sensitivity such that the infant's self-regulation capacities are facilitated. Another layer of complexity comes from the fact that many individual and family factors influence parents' ability to recognize and respond to their infant's discomfort and stress. Sensitive responding by the parent is affected by parental reflective functioning and psychological flexibility as well as parenting stress, parental mental health, parental experiences of abandonment, and parental history of exposure to ACEs. Finally, all the genetic, biological, and environmental factors that affect the path from parent–infant mutual coregulation to the infant's acquisition of a mature stress-regulation system are significantly influenced by family and community challenges (e.g., economic hardship, overcrowding, daily hassles, domestic and community violence, noise, pollution).[4-10]

Unrepaired Mismatches in Parent-Infan Coregulation

When *mismatches* in the parent–infant social-emotional relationship are highly frequent and typically not repaired, the infant has limited opportunities to develop and strengthen their stress-regulation system.[3,9] This is consequential as a less mature stress-regulation system results in the infant experiencing heightened sensitivity to stress and more frequent experiences of stress. Chronic stress leads to increasing dysregulation and disengagement, which may become permanently wired into neural circuitry as dysregulated rhythms in the autonomic nervous system. In addition, continued infant dysregulation requires the expenditure of high energy and interferes with the development of the infant's systems of arousal, emotions and behavior, and processes of healthy attachment.[3-4,8-10]

In sum, the roots of resilience are intertwined with the infant's development of a mature stress-regulation system that can manage stress, fear, and discomfort and make transitions from discomfort to well-being.[6,8,9] Sensitive and responsive parenting plays an important role in the healthy development of the infant's stress-regulation system. Both the need for sensitive and responsive parenting, such that the infant can manage stress and adversity, and the challenges to provide sensitive and responsive parenting are heightened in the context of poverty-related stressors and exposure to ACEs.[6–10]

Mindfulness and Mindfulness-Based Parenting Programs

Parents who adopt a mindfulness orientation for their parenting and regularly engage in mindful parenting practices will undergo a fundamental shift in their ability and willingness to truly be present with the constantly growing and changing nature of their child and their relationship with their child.

—Duncan, Coatsworth, and Greenberg[11]

Mindfulness and mindfulness meditation refer to psychological concepts and practices that have been associated with Buddhism and Buddhist psychology for more than 2,500 years. Mindfulness refers to the capacity for awareness, focused attention, nonreactivity to inner experience, and nonjudgmental acceptance of the present moment.[12,13] Consciousness associated with awareness, acceptance of the present moment, and low reactivity to unwanted thoughts stands in stark contrast to the frequent portrayal of modern life's consciousness with its automatic and unconscious avoidance of present-moment discomfort and reactive judgments of experiences, emotions, thoughts, and behaviors. Mindfulness meditation practices are designed to reorient attention to a more flexible awareness of the present moment and gentle acceptance of thoughts and discomfort. (See Box 10.1 for an illustration of one type of mindful meditation practice that supports awareness of the breath.) A more flexible, aware, and accepting consciousness is associated with higher well-being, self-compassion, and compassion for others.[13]

Mindfulness Based Interventions

Over the last 20 years, many cognitive-based clinical therapies have integrated the concepts of mindful awareness and practices of mindfulness meditation to increase the efficacy of treatments for adult depression, anxiety, stress, and PTSD.[13,14] Mindfulness-based stress reduction, the most well-known mindfulness-based intervention, has been shown to decrease stress, anxiety, and reactivity and increase coping ability in adults with chronic

---

Box 10.1. An Illustration of a Mindful Breathing Practice.

Sit comfortably with your feet on the floor and a straight spine and try to notice and follow your breath. Pay full attention to the sensations of your in-breath as it fills your lungs and your out-breath as it releases tension and leaves your body. When you recognize distraction and your thoughts have drifted away to thoughts about the future or the past, regain attentional focus to the present moment and pay full attention to your in-breath and out-breath with calm and curious acceptance of the experience.

---

pain. More specialized mindfulness-based interventions have been developed for treating addiction, severe depression, and other traumas, such as mindfulness-based relapse prevention, mindfulness-based cognitive therapy, acceptance and commitment therapy, dialectical behavior therapy, and mindful self-compassion.[13,14] A large body of rigorous evidence shows that there are physical and psychological health benefits of mindfulness-based interventions for adults who have experienced trauma.[13,15] In addition, the regular practice of mindfulness has been shown to have physical and psychological health benefits for healthy adults.[15] (See also chapter 3 by Shapiro and von Garnier in this volume.)

Mindful Parenting

Myla and Jon Kabat-Zinn's seminal book,[1] published in 1997 and entitled *Everyday Blessings: The Inner Work of Mindful Parenting*, proposed that a parental consciousness with full attention, emotional awareness, and acceptance supports many aspects of positive parenting, including parents' appreciation and compassion for their children, more thoughtful and nonreactive parental discipline strategies, and healthy parent–child attachment. They described mindfulness as creating a foundation for less reactivity during parenting challenges and more thoughtful and empathic overall parenting responses. The Kabat-Zinns' discussions regarding the benefits of nonreactive discipline and increased parental empathy aligned with a long history of work by attachment theorists who distinguished "sensitive" from "insensitive" caregiving in terms of higher levels of reflective functioning and stronger empathy for children.[16]

Researchers and practitioners have shown increasing interest in integrating concepts of mindful parenting into parent education programs.[11,17] Mindful parenting represents a shift from parenting programs focused primarily on behavior management to parenting programs connected more closely to healthy emotion regulation and healing parent–child relationships.[16] In 2009, the field was significantly advanced by Duncan, Coatsworth, and Greenberg,[11] who published a review of the empirical evidence for mindfulness and proposed a new and comprehensive model of mindful parenting. Their model included five critical foci of mindful parenting in the parent–child relationship: (1) listening with full attention, (2) full acceptance and nonjudgment of self and child, (3) emotional awareness of self and child, (4) self-regulation and emotion regulation in parent–child relationship, and (5) compassion for self and child. For each area of focus, Duncan and colleagues detailed the specific parenting behaviors that would be promoted and those that would be reduced by the practice of mindful parenting.

Bögels and Restifo[17] developed a mindful-parenting model grounded in mindfulness-based stress reduction and mindfulness-based cognitive therapy and published a session-by-session curriculum designed to treat parents, children, and youth with mental health problems. In Bögels and Restifo's model, mindful parenting positively addressed children's symptoms of psychopathology by affecting six aspects of parenting, including the reduction of the parent's stress and reactivity, the parent's focus on their child's psychopathology, and dysfunctional parenting habits. In addition, mindful parenting could be impactful by increasing the parent's executive functioning, parental self-care, and marital functioning and positive practices in coparenting. In addition to this model, Bögels and Restifo provided a guide for the cultivation of a personal mindfulness practice for health professionals.[17]

Efficacy of Mindfulness-Based Parenting Programs

Positive relationships among mindfulness, mindful parenting, and child outcomes have been found in nonclinical and clinical populations (ADHD, autism, developmental disabilities, etc.).[11,17] Researchers have demonstrated, with primarily correlational, case study, or small-scale designs, that mindful parenting practices are associated with decreases in parental stress and reactivity. Strong scientific evidence in support of MBPP is limited but growing. Some of the most rigorous evidence for MBPP has come from Coatsworth and colleagues,[18] who tested their model of mindful parenting using a randomized controlled trial (RCT). Their focus was on parenting during children's transition to adolescence, and in their intervention they integrated the mindful parenting model[11] with an established, empirically validated parent education program (i.e., Strengthening Families Program [SFP]: 10–14 years). Results showed that adding mindful parenting to SFP yielded significant and meaningful increases in multiple qualities of the parent–youth relationship. In a subsequent large-scale RCT of mindfulness-enhanced SFP: 10–14 (MSFP), Coatsworth and colleagues[19] confirmed their initial results and extended the analysis of MSFP to include mothers, fathers, and youth.

Bögels and Restifo's model[17] of mindful parenting was tested in a series of three controlled studies with families referred from child mental health centers. In each study, as predicted, they reported significant reductions in parental stress and overreactivity and increases in multiple aspects of mindful parenting. They also found reductions in both child and parent psychopathology symptoms.

Future work is needed to address limitations in the mindful-parenting literature. To advance the field of mindful parenting, studies must be conducted to evaluate specific ages of children, diagnoses for children, parent diagnoses, long-term follow-up, and different program curricula. Another limitation in the field is that there have been very few investigations of the mechanisms underlying the efficacy of MBPP. However, a recent paper by Laurent and colleagues[20] examined the efficacy of mindful parenting within a developmental psychobiological model and studied the relation of mindful parenting and both infants' and mothers' physiological responses to stress. They showed that the mother's management of physiological stress predicted the infant's responses and management of stress. Laurent and colleagues are the first researchers to provide physiological support for the idea that mindful parenting can act as a buffer against the experience of stress by the infant.

MBPPs for Families of Young Children Experiencing Adversity and Trauma

Mindfulness-based parenting programs emphasize reducing parental stress and reactivity and increasing parental capacities for nurturing and responsive caregiving. These emphases align with challenges faced by at-risk communities. The stressors and demands of parenting young children in disadvantaged communities are multiplied greatly due to challenges related to economic hardship, mental health, history of parental abandonment, overcrowding, work-related stresses, racial discrimination, and so on.[3-7,10] High levels of family and community stress may amplify challenges to parents' responsivity and psychological flexibility and thus negatively affect parents' capacity for sensitive responding to their infant's stress, fear, and discomfort. As described earlier, reduced parental capacity for sensitive caregiving is significant as unrepaired mismatches in the parent–infant social relationship impede the developmental path to mature infant stress regulation and self-regulation.[9] It is well established that nurturing, attentive, and attuned parenting supports the path from parent–infant mutual coregulation to infant self-regulation and profoundly affects the infant's developing brain and competencies that underlie resilience.[6-8,16]

Current knowledge about the developmental neurobiology of stress and the impact of nurturing environments suggests that MBPPs, with their emphasis on reducing parenting stress and reactivity and increasing nurturing caregiving, may be of particular benefit for families of young children experiencing adversity and trauma.[3–10,17–20]

Case Study: MBPP for Young Children Facing Adversity and Trauma

> When I take a couple minutes to relax and breathe with my baby in between daily chores, it helps my baby be more peaceful. I want to help protect my baby from the rough things going on in my neighborhood.
> —Participant in Safe, Secure and Loved (translated from Spanish)

Safe, Secure and Loved is a mindfulness-based parent support program designed to buffer the impact of poverty-related stressors, adversity, and trauma and promote resilience in young children. As shown in the schematic model in Figure 10.1, mindfulness and self-compassion practices, when combined with habits of resilience, support parent well-being and mindful family routines, and these competencies underlie children's trajectories of resilience.

We developed Safe, Secure and Loved using a modified implementation science framework[21] in a community facing extreme levels of adversity and trauma. The six-session group-based program introduces mindfulness and compassion practices as a way to promote responsive and nurturing parenting capacities that strengthen children's brain development and competencies of resilience.[22,23] Safe, Secure and Loved is organized around six habits of resilience that promote children's self-regulation, executive functioning, and secure attachment. Through guided discussion, role play, and family games, parents learn about the significance of nurturing and attentive parenting practices, family and community stressors, stress physiology and brain neuroplasticity, and healthy child development. Each habit of resilience is associated with a symbol (i.e., anchor, suitcase, heart, etc.), and parents complete a weekly craft as a home reminder for each symbol (i.e., anchor necklace, child's suitcase for future, compassionate heart pillow, etc.). Parents learn about the infant's stress-regulation system and explore ways to be more responsive, flexible, and aware during daily family routines in order to support brain development. Parents identify strategies to use the crafts to maintain more awareness during daily routines and unexpected challenges of their inner strengths, goals, values, and positive intentions for their children.

Beginning in 2013, in close partnership with a trauma-informed nonprofit agency that serves the Hispanic immigrant community, we started to pilot innovative ways to introduce, implement, and evaluate Safe, Secure and Loved. The program was offered in Spanish, and we enrolled Hispanic immigrant mothers with young children. Our assessments focused on parents' mental health and well-being, mindful awareness, and multiple aspects of positive parenting (e.g., family strengths, maternal confidence). Evaluations

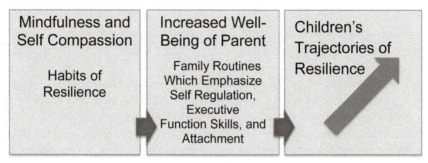

Figure 10.1 A Schematic Model of Safe Secure and Loved©. Practicing mindfulness and self compassion and habits of resilience support parental well-being and mindful family routines which emphasize young children's self regulation, executive functioning and secure attachment. These competencies underlie children's trajectories of resilience.

have shown consistent decreases in depression and increases in mindful awareness and multiple aspects of positive parenting. These findings are promising but limited by our use of single groups in pre-post designs with no comparison groups. Qualitative and anecdotal reports have revealed that parents readily adopt self-compassion practices and find mindfulness concepts beneficial and relevant to caregiving and broader family life. Participants talk about participation in Safe, Secure and Loved as a life-changing experience and share widely that the program has given them hope for themselves, their families, and their community. Following the completion of our very first parenting group, a large proportion of participants asked to continue their connection with the Safe, Secure and Loved program. This was unexpected. We responded to the community's strong motivation for continued engagement and identified ways to provide graduates of Safe, Secure and Loved opportunities to assist in facilitating future parent groups. In subsequent parent groups, this trend for graduates to stay connected to our program and volunteer to assist in future groups continued. We recognized the benefits of increased community engagement for widening the scale and sustainability of the program and using best practices from implementation science,[21] established, in partnership with our community agency, a formal training program for parents who were interested in becoming community champions.

Across a five-year period, the Safe, Secure and Loved program has transformed from a community-based MBPP to a *community-led* MBPP. In addition to manualized curricula for parents with young children at two ages (0–2 years and 3–5 years) and parent workbooks, we have a formal training program for community champions and fidelity protocols and procedures. In partnership with our nonprofit agency, parenting groups are now led by community champions at our original nonprofit as well as at schools, libraries, and faith-based institutions. We currently have more than 20 highly trained community champions, and we have enrolled more than 200 families.

The community response to our MBPP has been transformative for us as researchers and interventionists. We have identified several factors that appear to underlie this deep level of community engagement. First, the spiritual nature of mindful parenting seems to have provided a new and important dimension of parent education for families. Second, educating parents in mindfulness and compassion practices has allowed for more cultural variation in the adoption of resilience-strengthening parental behaviors, goals, and intentions. Third, having community champions lead the parent education program has increased the commitment to participation in the program. We believe that this transformation of Safe, Secure and Loved from a MBPP research intervention to a community-led MBPP program is significant as it demonstrates its potential to reach many more parents, support cultural variations of resilience, and promote community leaders. Currently, we are in the process of planning studies with larger samples such that we can implement a randomized controlled efficacy trial of our community-led MBPP.

Conclusions and Future Directions

> I believe that spirituality and science are complementary but different investigative approaches with the same goal of seeking the truth . . . there is much each may learn from the other, and together they may contribute to expanding the horizon of human knowledge and wisdom.
> —Fourteenth Dalai Lama[12]

Converging evidence from the neurobiology of stress, children's resilience, and clinical psychology underscores the significance of nurturing environments for children's social, emotional, and behavioral health. Promoting nurturing parenting practices is especially important for families of young children facing poverty-related stressors, adversity, and trauma. Mindfulness-based parenting programs, with their emphasis on simultaneously reducing parental stress and building on parents' inner strengths (e.g., reflective functioning, psychological flexibility, awareness) have great potential to support parental capacities to create more nurturing environments in culturally diverse communities. The early research on mindful parenting approaches has shown positive outcomes, including alleviation of parental stress and increased parental empathy, nurturing parenting practices, and positive child outcomes. The field, however, is at a very early stage. Few interventions have been empirically validated, and curricula and tools for implementation into community and clinical practice are not widely available.

Adoption of cultural strengths of resilience has been missing from many prevention and resilience-strengthening parenting programs. To support healing and strengthen resilience in communities experiencing adversity and trauma, developmental scientists and practitioners need to establish new ways to collaborate closely with the community and create more holistic interventions that build on the cultural variability of trajectories of resilience. The spiritual nature of mindful parenting interventions and the cultural relevance of resiliency have the potential to transcend barriers and establish parenting as community-driven primary prevention work.

References

1. Kabat-Zinn, M., & Kabat-Zinn, J. (1997). *Everyday blessings: The inner work of mindful parenting.* New York: Hyperion.

2. Felitti, V. J., Anda, R. F., Nordenberg, D., Williamson, D. F., Spitz, A. M., Edwards, V., . . . Marks, J. S. (1998). Relationship of childhood abuse and household dysfunction to many of the leading causes of death in adults: The adverse childhood experiences (ACE) study. *American Journal of Preventive Medicine, 14*(4), 245–258.

3. Osofsky, J. D., Stepka, P. T., & King, L. S. (2011). *Treating infants and young children impacted by trauma: Interventions that promote healthy development.* Washington, DC: American Psychological Association.

4. Gold, C. M. (2017). *The developmental science of early childhood.* New York: W. W. Norton & Co.

5. Shonkoff, J. P., Garner, A. S., Committee on Psychosocial Aspects of Child and Family Health, Committee on Early Childhood, Adoption, and Dependent Care, and Section on Developmental and Behavioral Pediatrics, Siegel, B. S., Dobbins, J. I., Earls, M. F., . . . Wood, D. L. (2012). The lifelong effects of early childhood adversity and toxic stress. *Pediatrics, 129,* 232–246.

6. National Scientific Council on the Developing Child. (2015). *Supportive relationships and active skill building strengthen the foundations of resilience.* Working Paper 13. Retrieved on March 12, 2018, from http://www.developingchild.harvard.edu

7. Masten, A. S. (2014). *Ordinary magic: Resilience in development.* New York: Guilford Press.

8. National Academies of Sciences, Engineering, and Medicine. (2016). *Parenting matters: Supporting parents of children ages 0–8.* Washington, DC: The National Academies Press. https://doi.org/10.17226/21868

9. Beeghly, M., & Tronick, E. (2011). Early resilience in the context of parent-infant relationships: A social developmental perspective. *Current Problems in Pediatric and Adolescent Health Care, 41,* 197–201.

10. Collins, K., Connors, K., Donohue, A., Gardner, S., Goldblatt, E., Hayward, A., . . . Thompson, E. (2010). *Understanding the impact of trauma and urban poverty on family systems: Risks, resilience and interventions.* Baltimore, MD: Family Informed Trauma Treatment Center. Retrieved from http://fittcenter .umaryland.edu/WhitPaper.aspx (link no longer active)

11. Duncan, L. G., Coatsworth, J. D., & Greenberg, M. T. (2009). A model of mindful parenting: Implications for parent-child relationships and prevention research. *Clinical Child and Family Psychology Review, 12*(3), 255–270.

12. Dalai Lama, H. H. (2005). *Essence of the heart sutra: The Dalai Lama's heart of wisdom teachings.* Somerville, MA: Wisdom.

13. Germer, C. K., Siegel, R. D., & Fulton, P. R. (Eds.). (2005). *Mindfulness and psychotherapy.* New York: Guilford Press.

14. Follette, V., Briere, J., Rozelle, D., Hopper, J. W., & Rome, D. I. *Mindfulness-oriented interventions for trauma: Integrating contemplative practices.* New York: Guilford Press.

15. Creswell, J. D. (2017). Mindfulness interventions. *Annual Review of Psychology, 68,* 18.1–18.26.

16. Burns, B. M., & Maritz, Y. (2015). Mindful Parents, Resilient Children: The Significance of Compassion for Parenting. *The Psychology of Compassion and Cruelty: Understanding the Emotional, Spiritual, and Religious Influences: Understanding the Emotional, Spiritual, and Religious Influences* (pp. 125–142), Santa Barbara, CA: ABC-CLIO.

17. Bögels, S. M., & Restifo, K. (2014). *Mindful parenting: A guide for mental health practitioners.* New York: Springer.

18. Coatsworth, J. D., Duncan, L. G., Greenberg, M. T., & Nix, R. L. (2010). Changing parents' mindfulness, child management skills and relationship quality with their youth: Results from a randomized pilot intervention trial. *Journal of Child and Family Studies, 19,* 203–217.

19. Coatsworth, J. D., Duncan, L. G., Nix, R. L., Greenberg, M., Gayles, J. G., Bamberger, K. T., . . . Demi, M. A. (2015). Integrating mindfulness with parent training: Effects of the Mindfulness-Enhanced Strengthening Families Program. *Developmental Psychology, 51*(1), 26–35.

20. Laurent, H. K., Duncan, L. G., Lightcap, A., & Khan, F. (2017). Mindful parenting predicts mothers' and infants' hypothalamic-pituitary adrenal activity during a dyadic stressor. *Developmental Psychology, 53*(3), 47–424.

21. Metz, A., Naoom, S. F., Halle, R., & Bartley, L. (2015). *An integrated stage-based framework for implementation of early childhood programs and systems (OPRE 201548).* Washington, DC: US DHHS.

22. Burns, B., Haynes, L., Bauer, A., Shetty, A., Mendoza, J., Fregoso, F., . . . Arellano, B. (2013). Strengthening children's resilience through parenting: A pilot study. *Therapeutic Communities: International Journal of Therapeutic Communities, 34*(4), 121–131.

23. Burns, B. M., Fayram, E., Strong, K., Ruiz, A., Arellano, B., Ilcicin, M., . . . Vaccaro, J. (2015). The resilient families program: Promoting children's resilience through parenting. *Wheelock International Journal of Children, Families, and Social Change, 1*(1), e1–e10.

CHAPTER ELEVEN

Promoting Hope, Healing, and Wellness: Catholic Interventions in Behavioral Health Care

Thomas G. Plante and Gerdenio (Sonny) Manuel, S.J.

The Catholic Church includes over a billion people and is the largest single church denomination in the United States, representing approximately 23 percent of the total U.S. population.[1,2] It is the oldest continuous organization of any kind in the world with a 2,000-plus-year history. Furthermore, the Catholic Church, via its various religious orders of priests, religious sisters and brothers, and lay colleagues, as well as the sponsorship of numerous dioceses, operates countless private schools at the elementary, secondary, and collegiate levels across the country and around the world. Additionally, they direct hospitals and social service agencies in many countries around the world.[1] Regardless of one's religious background, tradition, or beliefs, Catholic or otherwise, numerous lives are being, or have been, significantly affected by the Catholic Church through education, medical care, social services, and pastoral support.

Health-care professionals are likely to treat Catholics; and many of these professionals, regardless of their own religious or spiritual affiliations, work in Catholic-affiliated institutions. It is, therefore, important for these professionals to better understand this religious tradition and appreciate the hope and healing this tradition may offer them and their clients or patients. Research and clinical best practices have found that many Catholic spiritual practices and rituals can be well integrated into treatment approaches in successful ways.[3,4] Many of these strategies may not be completely unique to Catholicism but are also accepted and shared by other faith traditions. For example, prayer, meditation, religious rituals, sacred music, and so forth are vital practices for many different faith traditions.[5-8]

Over the centuries that Catholic faith and spirituality evolved, a long list of religious and spiritual practices engaged the faithful, promising help for them and their loved ones as they coped with various physical and psychological ailments, stressors, and concerns. These practices include, in part, prayer, meditation, anointing, Mass attendance, other special ritual experiences, community service (particularly with the poor, marginalized, and challenged), modeling and following the examples of Jesus and the saints, and so forth.[1,9] Until recently, most of these religious and spiritual strategies haven't been subjected to rigorous outcome research or clinical trials or incorporated into any evidence-based professional practice protocols. While a great deal of research still needs to be done, a wide variety of scholars and practitioners have addressed the integration of religious and spiritual practices in evidence-based ways.[3,6,7] Often this work has been undertaken in the spirit of multicultural competency training encouraging evidence-based treatment interventions that fit clients and their patient diversity profiles, including those based on gender, ethnicity, race, sexual orientation, and religion.[10] In fact, the American Psychological Association's code of ethics actually demands that professional psychologists respect and attend to diversity issues, including those based on religious diversity.[11]

In this chapter, we will outline, highlight, and review some of the Catholic traditions and pastoral tools that can be integrated into any professional clinical practice in behavioral health care. We will focus our attention on six tools in particular that are particularly popular and unique within the Catholic faith tradition. We will also offer brief case illustrations to provide examples of how these Catholic tools can be effectively integrated into professional clinical practice.

Prayer

Prayer is often defined as a conversation or contemplative encounter with the divine or sacred, a practice supported by all major religious traditions. Research has found that prayer enhances psychological health, stress management, and coping,[7,12] as well as physical health.[13]

Catholic tradition includes prayers common to many Christian denominations and traditions (e.g., the Our Father or the Lord's Prayer, the Jesus

Prayer, the Prayer of St. Francis) as well as those more uniquely suited to Catholic populations (e.g., the Hail Mary, the Rosary). For those who are not familiar with the aforementioned most popular prayers, they are offered here:

The Lord's Prayer

(Matt. 6:9–13)

Our Father in heaven, hallowed be Your name.
Your kingdom come, Your will be done, on earth as it is in heaven.
Give us this day our daily bread, and forgive us our debts,
as we also have forgiven our debtors.
And lead us not into temptation, but deliver us from evil.
For Yours is the kingdom, the power and the glory forevermore.
Amen.

The Hail Mary

Hail Mary full of Grace, the Lord is with thee.
Blessed are thou among women and blessed is the fruit of thy womb, Jesus.
Holy Mary Mother of God, pray for us sinners now and
at the hour of our death.
Amen.

The Jesus Prayer

Lord Jesus Christ, Son of God, have mercy on me, a sinner.

In additional to these ritualized and specific prayers, spontaneous prayers (like intentions, petitions, and simple conversations with God, Jesus, Mary, and the saints) are prevalent within the Catholic tradition as they often are in various religious traditions and denominations.

Prayer can help clients and patients feel better, organizing and centering them as their prayer binds their anxiety and fear and offers them hope. Prayer can be a powerful reminder that they are not alone in their suffering and that God is with them—offering them forgiveness, deliverance, mercy, and compassion as reflected upon in the aforementioned prayers. Prayer connects them to a tradition, community, and belief system that expands their horizons and helps them see beyond themselves. Prayer practices can be easily integrated into psychotherapy and self-help strategies for coping and managing a wide variety of mental and physical health challenges.[3,6]

Case Example 1: Bob

Bob is a middle-aged, married, successful Silicon Valley executive who has worked for some of the top technology companies in the area. He is Catholic, though his wife is an Episcopalian. Both are interested and engaged in their respective religious denominations, which they describe as more similar than not.

Bob struggles with anger management and an obsessive-compulsive personality disorder. He can fly off the handle when things don't go his way, and he often feels guilty about his reactions to the many frustrations associated with his marriage and work.

Wanting to integrate his faith and religious tradition into his psychotherapy, he agreed to work with a spiritual director to complement the work of his therapist. He started to use the Jesus Prayer as a mantra, praying it over and over throughout the day and most especially when he felt vulnerable in situations that triggered his frustration and anger. Additionally, he would recite the Hail Mary when he tried to sleep and when he found himself obsessing about matters of the day. These prayers helped break the escalating associations that fuel his frustration, anger, and rumination. He explained that praying reminded him of what is important and put his troubles in a larger context. "It was comforting to know that I was not alone with my anxiety and frustration, that God was present and offered me understanding and compassion." Being attentive to his faith and religious community helped him to become still and stay calm.

Meditation

All religious traditions offer strategies for contemplation and meditation, which have seen a recent explosion of research examining their effectiveness.[14–16] During the past decade or so, mindfulness meditation has attracted the most intense interest in both practice and research. Although originating within the Buddhist tradition, mindfulness has been secularized so that it is welcomed in both diverse religious and secular communities.[15,17] Many contemporary mindfulness practitioners likely have no sense that this approach to meditation has a religious foundation at all.

The Catholic tradition offers variations on this popular meditative approach, such as centering prayer. Developed and popularized during the 1960s and 1970s by Trappist monks Thomas Keating and Thomas Merton,[18,19] centering prayer and meditation can amplify other kinds of prayer. Practitioners explain that "it adds depth of meaning to all prayer and facilitates the movement from more active modes of prayer—verbal, mental or affective prayer into a receptive prayer of resting in God."[20] Similarly, other meditative practices have been developed by the Catholic tradition (e.g., Eucharist adoration, novenas, Lectio Divina) as well, too numerous to detail here, that highlight the intimacy and power of one's personal relationship with God, a relationship that can surpass words and move from conversation to communion. One especially popular approach "to find God in all things" originates in the spiritual exercises of St. Ignatius,[21,22] which include discovery, detachment, discernment, and direction, which culminate in a final meditation on how God loves without limit and how that love can grow in the hearts and lives of those who engage in these spiritual exercises.[4,21–23] Like mindfulness, many of the Catholic-influenced meditative approaches have been adapted to appeal to those who might not share the Catholic tradition.

Case Example 2: Beth

Beth is a divorced woman in her early seventies. She adopted three children at birth, who are now all young adults. Sadly, unbeknownst to her, each of the children was drug exposed in the womb, and now all suffer from the consequences of fetal alcohol syndrome as well as other related ailments. She is often sick with fear about her adult children, who live generally marginalized and self-destructive lives, making reckless decisions that she finds exasperating. As a lifelong Catholic who now attends an Episcopalian church, she finds comfort and some solace through centering prayer techniques. She explains that when she cannot find the words to convey the depth of her fear for her children, or finds herself exhausted by her lamentations, she can turn to centering prayer to rest in God. She experiences this prayer as a way of being held silently by God even as she is powerless to change the circumstances of her children.

Mass

Rituals can be found within all major religious and spiritual traditions. The Eucharist, or more popularly "the Mass," is perhaps the most well-known and important of the Catholic rituals. The Eucharist is a liturgy of thanksgiving recalling Jewish table blessings that highlight how God is at work in the human community and all of creation.[24,25] It recalls particularly the Last Supper, or the Passover meal that Jesus shared with his disciples before he died, where he broke bread and shared wine, pledging, "This is my body, given up for you." This liturgy of the Eucharist or thanksgiving includes biblical readings, a brief sermon or homily, a variety of special prayers, and Holy Communion; at Mass, Catholics believe they are fed both by the word of God and the body of the Lord in the reception of the bread and wine and in the community gathered around them.

At Mass, Catholics celebrate in thanksgiving that they are not alone or abandoned but seen, felt, touched, fed, and solaced by God and their faith community living and dead, here and now, and forever joined no matter what the future might bring. Thus, "every time this mystery is celebrated, 'the work of our redemption is carried on' and we 'break the one bread that provides the medicine of immortality, the antidote for death, and the food that makes us live forever in Jesus Christ.'"[24,25]

A deeply contemplative and prayerful experience, the Mass is often cele-brated in a typically lovely and sacred church environment featuring reli-gious icons and art and accompanied by inspiring and meditative religious hymns and music. Mass can be a centering and organizing time and practice for attendees, providing a feeling of safety and security and calling them forth to become part of something bigger and more sacred than the solitary self. It can be an occasion to deepen awareness of and commitment to the action of God in a person's life and community at every moment. Engage-ment with other Mass attendees also allows for social support and involve-ment with those of like mind, interest, and faith.

Case Example 3: Martin and Maria

Martin and Maria have been happily married for 35 years and enjoy the company of their four grown children, two of whom are recently married and have given them their first grandchildren. Recently retired, Martin has been looking forward to traveling the world with Maria and spending more time with his children and grandchildren. One year into Martin's retirement, Maria and Martin discover that Maria's breast cancer has returned. They are devastated and worried; neither can imagine life without the other. As Maria begins treatment, they find hope and encouragement from attending Mass together daily. They explain how they find that within the Mass they can pray together for Maria's healing but are also consoled by how God's word reminds them of their blessings and gives them courage to face whatever the day brings. Receiving communion deepens their sense of connection not only to one another but also to their family and friends. Maria and Martin, fed by God's word and the Eucharist of bread and wine, are consoled by God's promise of eternal love and by the idea that their own love is forever joined to God—whatever the future might bring. They cannot imagine how they could manage these months of uncertainly without the comfort, cour-age, and connection they experience together at Mass.

Confession

The Catholic tradition offers the faithful another healing and solacing rit-ual, "the sacrament of reconciliation," popularly known as confession, to experience "not simply reconciliation with God, but with all human forms of reconciliation, whether intrapsychic or interpersonal, whether between members of families or between whole communities; the Catholic rite of rec-onciliation is intended as a paradigm for all human reconciliation."[26] Within the ritual, penitents can talk with a priest about their troubles, confessing their sins and acknowledging how their actions have hurt others and them-selves. The priest may respond with some limited pastoral counseling followed by prayers and absolution (i.e., explicit forgiveness of their sins) and end by suggesting a penance that typically involves an act of restorative justice and/or a recitation of traditional prayers, such as Our Fathers and Hail Marys.[9] Although not as popular within Western culture now as in the past, confession is an important staple of Catholic life.

Whatever is stated or confessed during this sacrament is held in strict confidence, as priests are not mandated reporters when it comes to child abuse, danger to self and others, and so on when they learn of these issues through the confessional experience. Catholics often report feeling relieved after confessing to a priest, knowing that what they say is held in strict confidence. In addition, they can engage the ritual of confession in a completely anonymous manner by using traditional confessionals, private rooms or booths in Catholic churches. These confessionals are designed to protect confidentiality in that the priest and the penitent cannot see each other and speak through a "window" that is usually very small and often opaque.

Confession is now also offered face to face in a church office setting. In this way, confession is no longer "anonymous"; the priest and penitent can see each other without obstruction. What is voiced during confession, however, remains completely confidential. This more modern venue allows for conversation, spiritual advising, and direction in a more natural, personal environment. Priests report that much of confession becomes pastoral counseling and advising in these settings as well. The actual act of confession of sins is often a brief part of the overall encounter where pastoral care and spiritual discussion and problem solving takes the bulk of the time.

Case Example 4: Lena

Lena is a devout Catholic in her forties who had a brief marital affair. She has a long history of anxiety, experiencing separation anxiety as a child and panic attacks along with agoraphobia as an adult. She has always struggled with feelings of guilt about many issues. Her brief marital affair never resulted in sexual intercourse but included flirtation, kissing, and fondling. After the affair was over, she felt intensely guilty, which decreased the gains that she had made in managing her anxiety disorder. She could not bring herself to tell her husband, believing that such an out-of-character revelation might cause irreparable damage to their relationship. The consequences of her sin were threats to her identity and the loss of her personal freedom and power, which resulted in deep feelings of social isolation and interpersonal alienation. Her panic attacks increased significantly, and she felt more and more anxious and agoraphobic.

After confessing to her parish priest, she felt much better for some time, and through engaging the acts of penance mandated by her confession, she began to feel healed of her estrangement from herself and her husband.

However, after several years, she felt that she needed a "booster" session and returned to confession to admit her sin of marital infidelity once again. During the second confessional experience, the priest suggested that she engage in ongoing pastoral counseling in addition to her psychotherapy, and she gladly accepted his advice. Confession and pastoral care along with her psychotherapy became an important part of her efforts to better manage her guilt and anxiety.

The Saints

Catholics have a long list of saints, and many days of the year are designated feast days for one or more of them.[9] Saints typically act as spiritual models who reflect a devout life of prayer, good works, and strong faith. Saints include men and women, some of very high rank, such as previous popes, and others who are peasants or even children.[27] Many were martyred or suffered violently due to their beliefs or saintly actions. Church-related schools, colleges, parishes, and other houses of worship and retreat centers are often named after saints, and many cities, towns, and even a state are named after saints as well (e.g., San Francisco, St. Louis, San Jose, Maryland). While some Catholics pray to the saints for intercessions and have particular prayers associated with each one, most importantly saints provide a narrative of a life well lived, patterned after Christ and witnessing to their faith through action.

Research on observational learning[28–30] makes clear that people learn from watching the behavior of others. Bandura offers a four-step process of effective observational learning that includes attention, retention, reproduction, and motivation. In other words, people are asked to attend to the model of interest, remember what they did and said, reproduce their behavior, and then work to motivate themselves to continue doing so. Appealing models are highlighted, and people are encouraged to follow them. The popular question "What would Jesus do?" (often referred to as WWJD) is an excellent example. The famous Good Samaritan parable from the Gospel of Luke (Luke 10:25–37) ends with the command, "Go and do likewise."

Stories about Jesus, his disciples, and the numerous saints throughout the ages provide rich material to work with in helping those with mental and physical health problems find role models who inspire hope and healing. Effective strategies for coping can be found among the numerous examples of these important religious figures.[27,28]

Case Example 1: Bob

Bob, from the example presented earlier, often feels very guilty about his thoughts and behaviors that are a by-product of his obsessive-compulsive personality. He often struggles with feeling sinful and gets frustrated that he can't adequately control his thoughts and behaviors. He worries that his sinfulness may be religiously damming, and his frustration results in angry outbursts, making his feelings and worries even worse. However, Bob takes solace in reflecting on the impulsivity of St. Peter as well as Jesus's own anger when he overturned the tables in the temple, which many theologians point to as the reason local authorities decided to find a way to kill him (Matt. 21:12–17). In addition, Saint Mother Teresa of Calcutta is a model for him as her spiritual doubts are well articulated in her autobiography even as she remained faithful to her life of simplicity and service.[31] Bob finds comfort in reflecting on her story of managing and coping with religious questions and spiritual dryness. In the company of these and other saints, Bob feels more relaxed and accepting of his own humanity and still inspired to pursue more healthy behavior and thinking.

Charitable Service

Finally, most religious and spiritual traditions focus attention on service to others and especially those who struggle in some important way. These others include the poor, homeless, elderly, refugees, the sick and despairing, and other people in great need. Catholic groups run countless soup kitchens, food pantries, relief services both domestic and international, and hospitals and clinics for those who are indigent. While these charitable works are commonly practiced among numerous religious and spiritual groups, Catholics, due to their long history, large numbers, and many religious communities of nuns and priests who specialize in particular charitable or service activities (e.g., Mother Teresa's Missionaries of Charity, Society of St. Vincent de Paul), offer many unique opportunities for service engagement across the globe.

Research finds that volunteer and service activities benefit not only others but also the helpers themselves. Helping others while engaging in volunteerism, community-based interventions, and the like enhances stress management, self-esteem, and compassion and is even associated with increased longevity.[32–34] These opportunities help those who are distressed move out of their narrow window of challenges, assist other people, feel good about their efforts, and enhance their self-efficacy as well.

Case Example 5: Larry

Larry is an elderly man who never married, never had children, and as an only child, he didn't have siblings or nieces and nephews either. His parents have passed away, and he has no known relatives. After retiring as an engineer, he got involved in the St. Vincent de Paul Society at his parish; the society's mission is to offer hope and service through direct person-to-person contact. He was reluctant at first, but as he got to know the other volunteers and the clients, he became more and more engaged in their activities and also donated a significant amount of money to causes helping those most in need. Larry has a history of depression as well as some struggles with fibromyalgia. He can isolate himself due to his mental and physical health problems. Yet, his volunteer activities moved him to connect with others and engage in the good works of St. Vincent de Paul on a regular basis. His large donations have been well received and provide appreciated attention from not only the society and his parish but also from the bishop of the diocese. Recently he was asked to serve on the board of directors for the national organization. He freely admits that he gets more out of his volunteer activities than he gives, describing them as a form of self-help, a life-changing activity that has resulted in lasting behavioral and attitudinal change as he finds himself less worried about himself and more engaged by helping others. His service connects him to a faith that he finds deeply sustaining, as his faith moves him to build relationships that are ultimately healing.

Conclusion

The Roman Catholic Church has survived and thrived for over 2,000 years and over time developed a wide range of spiritual and religious practices in the service of helping the faithful live a healthy and holy life. Research has confirmed that these practices help manage the stressors and challenges of life. They can be integrated into psychotherapy and help treat both physical and mental health troubles and challenges. Many of these strategies have been adapted for use with non-Catholics as well with some being secularized in ways that can appeal to people of all religious faiths or even no religious faith.

Additional research that uses the state-of-the-art methodological strategies of randomized clinical trials is much needed to adequately determine the effectiveness of Catholic spiritual and religious interventions in behavioral health care. Investigators should be encouraged and supported for engaging in this research as well. In the meantime, preliminary research evidence and best clinical practices seem to suggest that Catholic religious and spiritual strategies that include prayer, meditation, Mass attendance, confession and reconciliation, modeling the lives of the saints, and service to the community among others can be professionally and effectively utilized in behavioral health services. In addition, in the spirit of multiculturalism and respect for diversity (including religious diversity), engaging Catholic clients and patients in psychotherapy and both mental and physical health care by being respectful of and welcoming of their unique spiritual and religious tradition is important and recommended.

References

1. Allen, J. L. (2009). *The future church: How ten trends are revolutionizing the Catholic Church.* New York: Random House.

2. Pew Forum on Religion and Public Life. (2008). *United States religious landscape survey: Religious affiliation—diversity & dynamics.* Washington, DC: Author.

3. Plante, T. G. (2009). *Spiritual practices in psychotherapy: Thirteen tools for enhancing psychological health.* Washington, DC: American Psychological Association.

4. Plante, T. G. (2017). The 4 Ds: Using Ignatian spirituality in secular psychotherapy and beyond. *Spirituality in Clinical Practice, 4*(1), 74–79.

5. McCullough, M. E., & Larson, D. B. (1999). Prayer. In W. R. Miller (Ed.), *Integrating spirituality into treatment* (pp. 85–110). Washington, DC: American Psychological Association.

6. Pargament, K. I. (2007). *Spiritually integrated psychotherapy: Understanding and addressing the sacred.* New York: Guilford Press.

7. Pargament, K., Exline, J., Jones, J., Mahoney, A., & Shafranske, E. (2013). *APA handbooks in psychology: APA handbook of psychology, religion, and spirituality.* Washington, DC: American Psychological Association.

8. Sanders, P. W., Richards, P. S., McBride, J. A., Lea, T., Hardman, R. K., & Barnes, D. V. (2015). Processes and outcomes of theistic spiritually oriented psychotherapy: A practice-based evidence investigation. *Spirituality in Clinical Practice, 2*(3), 180.

9. Catholic Church. (2000). *Catechism of the Catholic Church* (No. 5–109). Washington, DC: United States Conference of Catholic Bishops Publishing.

10. Plante, T. G. (2014). Four steps to improve religious/spiritual competence in professional psychology. *Spirituality in Clinical Practice, 1*(4), 288–292.

11. American Psychological Association. (2002). Ethical principles of psychologists and code of conduct. *American Psychologist, 57,* 1060–1073.

12. Richards, P. S., & Bergin, A. E. (2005). *A spiritual strategy for counseling and psychotherapy* (2nd ed.). Washington, DC: American Psychological Association.

13. Koenig, H. G., McCullough, M. E., & Larson, D. B. (2001). *Handbook of religion and health.* New York: Oxford University Press.

14. Gemer, C. K., Siegel, R. D., & Fulton, P. R. (Eds.). (2013). *Mindfulness and psychotherapy.* New York: Guilford Press.

15. Kabat-Zinn, J. (2003). Mindfulness-based interventions in context: Past, present, and future. *Clinical Psychology: Research and Practice, 10,* 144–156.

16. Plante, T. G. (2016). Beyond mindfulness: Expanding integration of spirituality and religion into psychotherapy. *Open Theology, 2,* 135–144.

17. Kabat-Zinn, J. (1994). *Wherever you go, there you are.* New York: Hyperion.

18. Keating, T. (1981). *The heart of the world: An introduction to contemplative Christianity.* New York: Crossroad Publishing.

19. Merton, T. (1973). *Contemplation in a world of action.* Garden City: Image Books.

20. Keating, T. (n.d.). Centering prayer. In *Centering prayer: Silence solitude simplicity and service.* Retrieved on March 12, 2018, from http://www.contempla tiveoutreachireland.com/centering-prayer/

21. Mottola, A. (Trans.). (1964). *The spiritual exercises of St. Ignatius: St. Ignatius' profound precepts of mystical theology.* New York: Doubleday.

22. Olin, J. C. (Ed.). (1992). *The autobiography of St. Ignatius Loyola* (J. F. O'Callahan, Trans.). New York: Fordham.

23. Dreher, D. E., & Plante, T. G. (2007). Rediscovering the sense of calling: Promoting greater health, joy, and purpose in life. In T. G. Plante & C. E. Thoresen (Eds.), *Spirit, science and health: How the spiritual mind fuels physical wellness* (pp. 129–142). Westport, CT: Praeger/Greenwood.

24. Catholic Church. (2017a). The Eucharist—pledge of the glory to come. In *Catechism of the Catholic Church* (1405) (2nd ed.). Vatican City: Libreria Editrice Vaticana.

25. Catholic Church. (2017b). The sacrament of the Eucharist—the sacramental sacrifice thanksgiving, memorial, presence. In *Catechism of the Catholic Church* (1362–1365) (2nd ed.). Vatican City: Libreria Editrice Vaticana.

26. Kiesling, C. (1970). Paradigms of sacramentality. *Worship, 44*(7), 426.

27. Martin, J. (2007). *My life with the saints.* Chicago, IL: Loyola.

28. Bandura, A. (2003). On the psychosocial impact and mechanisms of spiritual modeling. *The International Journal for the Psychology of Religion, 13,* 167–174.

29. Bandura, A. (1997). *Self-efficacy: The exercise of control.* New York: W. H. Freeman.

30. Bandura, A. (1986). *Social foundations of thought and action: A social cognitive theory.* Englewood Cliffs, NJ: Prentice Hall.

31. Mother Teresa. (2007). *Come be my light: The private writings of the "Saint of Calcutta"* (B. Kolodiejchuk, Ed.). New York: Random House.

32. Harris, A. H., & Thoresen, C. E. (2005). Volunteering is associated with delayed mortality in older people: Analysis of the longitudinal study of aging. *Journal of Health Psychology, 10*(6), 739–752.

33. Mills, B. A., Bersamina, R. B., & Plante, T. G. (2007). The impact of college student immersion service learning trips on coping with stress and vocational identity. *The Journal for Civic Commitment, 9,* 1–8.

34. Plante, T. G., & Halman, K. E. (2016). Nurturing compassion development among college students: A longitudinal study. *Journal of College and Character, 17*(3), 164–173.

CHAPTER TWELVE

Holistic Healing in Eastern Orthodox Christianity

John T. Chirban

Healing in Eastern Orthodox Christianity traces back to the ministry of Jesus Christ. Jesus returned to Nazareth and read from the prophesy of Isaiah:

> The Spirit of the Lord is upon me,
> Because the Lord has anointed me to preach good news to the poor.
> He has sent me to proclaim release to the captives.
> And recovering of sight to the blind.
> To set at liberty those who are oppressed
> To proclaim the acceptable year of the Lord. (Luke 4:18–19)

Christ's approach to his healing mission is founded on the Hebraic holistic notion of personhood—an understanding preserved by the church fathers, practiced in the Byzantine Empire (since 330 CE), and retained by Eastern Orthodox Christianity to the present day. Numerous prominent religious leaders within Eastern Orthodox Christianity were both physicians and spiritual leaders. SS Kosmas and Damian,[1] Basil the Great, and Photios were among those who made significant contributions to healing, demonstrating the Christian affirmation for growing in wholeness.[2]

This paper describes the holistic epistemology of Eastern Orthodox Christianity concerning healing and identifies practices of healing by the Orthodox Christian faithful that remain to this day.

Jesus Christ as Healer

The ministry of Jesus Christ involves restoring, curing, and making a person whole: healing body, mind, and soul. The Gospel of Matthew (9:35) reports Christ's miraculous interventions: "Jesus went about . . . healing all manner of sickness and all manner of disease among the people." He cured people of physical, emotional, and spiritual maladies, and he encouraged wholeness through spiritual awakening. Both rabbi and preacher, Jesus affirmed his authority to heal as the Son of Man (Matt. 16:13–16) and the Son of God (Luke 22:70), as well as the purpose for which the Gospel of John is written (John 20:31). Christ's ministry of healing explains what health truly is.

Responding to pleas for relief from physical and emotional agony, Jesus described an essential spiritual core as the basis for health. Even as Jesus cured physical dysfunction with diverse interventions, he circled back to a spiritual message. With his awareness of human nature, health, and illness, he treated healing as a psychosomatic phenomenon. In numerous instances when he healed blindness, reports explain that Christ invoked different interventions, conveying different resources as agents for the healing process.

In one instance, Jesus cured blindness by placing spit on a blind man's eyes and then laying his hands upon them (John 9:6). The man still did not see, so Jesus touched the man's eyes and directed him to look upward, at which point the man was healed. Here, a salient element for healing appears to be the person's active participation.

"Two blind men followed him, calling out, 'Have mercy on us, Son of David!' When he had gone indoors, the blind men came to him, and he asked them, 'Do you believe that I am able to do this?' 'Yes, Lord,' they replied. Then he touched their eyes and said, 'According to your faith let it be done to you'" (Matt. 9:27–29). In this instance, their faith in Christ cures them.

Later,

> As Jesus and his disciples were leaving Jericho, a large crowd followed him. Two blind men were sitting by the roadside, and when they heard Jesus going by, they shouted, "Lord, Son of David, have mercy on us!" The crowd rebuked them, but they shouted louder, "Lord, Son of David, have mercy on us!" Jesus called to them. "What do you want me to do for you?" he asked. "Lord," they answered, "we want our sight." Jesus had compassion on them and touched their eyes. Immediately they received their sight and followed him. (Matt. 20:29–34)

These healings appear connected to the faith of the recipients and Christ's compassion.

With the blind man at Siloam, Jesus spit in the dust, made a clay paste with the saliva, rubbed the paste on the blind man's eyes, and said, "Go, wash at the Pool of Siloam." The man washed and saw (John 9:6–7). In this case, Christ focused on a specific physical intervention and engaged the man's active involvement.

In Mark 8:23–26:

> He took the blind man by the hand, and led him outside the village. When he had spit on his eyes and put his hands upon him, Jesus asked him if he saw. He looked up and said, "I see people; they look like trees walking around." Once more Jesus put his hands on the man's eyes. Then his eyes were opened, his sight was restored, and he saw everything clearly.

In this situation, attunement and refinement of treatment occurs in the intervention.

Christ also responded to "the source" for blindness: "And his disciples asked him, saying, 'Rabbi, who sinned, this man or his parents, that he was born blind?' Jesus answered, 'Neither this man or his parents sinned: but this happened so that the works of God might be made manifest in him'" (John 9:2–3). In this instance, revelatory significance provides the explanation for blindness.

The prophecy of Isaiah that Christ read about his "recovering sight to the blind" was revealed through his ministry as both an ability to cure physical deficits and to remedy humanity's deeper spiritual darkness: "Though seeing they do not see" (Matt. 13:13). "That seeing they may see" (Mark 4:12).

Eastern Orthodox Christianity

Based on Christ's understanding of the interdependent nature of personhood (body, mind, and soul), Eastern Orthodox Christians approached healing holistically. Emphasizing the importance and synergy of the healing disciplines, early Eastern Orthodox Christians or Byzantines (330–1453 CE) integrated religious rituals with medical treatment, believing that patients would obtain full health when connected to God and the church community. In Eastern Orthodox Christianity, healers also distinguished specializations in view of primary professional functions (e.g., clergy, nun, or physician). Frequently, both roles were combined to attend to healing and caring for the whole person.

In the fourth century, Byzantine institutions began to focus on curing the sick. Hospitals were often built near churches, which were recognized as appropriate locations for the faithful to find physical, emotional, and spiritual care. Both priests and medical doctors offered treatment. The Byzantines saw a direct correlation between the sickness of the body and the sickness of the soul.[3] Byzantine medical professionals developed clinical procedures, pharmacology, and surgery. Many of their innovations remain today. Among Byzantine medical advances were diagnostic orthopedic devices for healing fractures and for performing angio-aneurysms, hysterectomies, craniotomies, tonsillectomies, mastectomies, and tracheotomies, as well as diagnostic techniques for arteriosclerosis, blood viscosity, endocarditis, pericarditis, and dozens more.[4]

Psychosomatic Epistemology and Methodologies of Healing

The Eastern Orthodox Christian understanding of healing is faith based yet embraces science. As Byzantine physicians made connections between science and human functioning, these discoveries raised further questions about the nature of the soul.[5] Byzantine science exercised powerful influence on the patristic tradition that encouraged reason as a way to truth guided by faith. The interdependence of the separate domains of faith and science were formative to the development of Byzantine psychosomatic epistemology.

Numerous individual approaches for healing have existed within the integrative, psychosomatic epistemology of Orthodox Christian practice. Based on the range of evidence of the psychosomatic epistemology, six primary methodologies emerge:[6]

1. Rational methodologies
2. Moral methodologies
3. Affective methodologies
4. Experiential methodologies
5. Ontological methodologies
6. Connatural methodologies

These discrete categories are not necessarily exclusive, as a given healer may utilize several approaches. At the same time, it is important to recognize that there is not one single Orthodox methodological perspective. In fact, numerous methodologies convey both diverse and conflicting methodologies, though they are unified by affirmation of central tenets of faith.[7]

1. Rational methodologies: Many church fathers wrote about the importance of the rational processes as a means for achieving a healthy mind, body, and spirit and as a vehicle to know God. The antipathy between those who pursued the "scientific" disciplines and those with church professions occur most frequently at the fringes of disciplines in Eastern Christianity. Expressing the central theological stance in the East, St. Basil wrote, "The mind is a wonderful thing."[8] Rational processes were understood as essential steps on the path toward true knowledge, not ends in themselves. In conjunction with rational methodology, it was recognized that God empowered humanity with the autonomous power to heal body, mind, and soul, and that rational faculties are a gateway to specific interventions for healing.[9]

2. Moral methodologies: The moral approach associates direct and indirect correlation of physical health and "moral hygiene." Both righteous and sinful behavior affects wellness, but there is no direct correlation. An example of the connection between living a moral and virtuous life and health is found in "The Miracles of St. Photeine," a hagiography from the 11th to 12th century, in which a man is said to be stricken with blindness for having "a lustful eye."[10] Morality and spiritual affliction may engender a psychosomatic response in these instances. Modern psychological studies confirm that emotional and physical illness may derive from existential or spiritual problems.[11] At the same time, St. Diadochos cautioned his Christian readers not to boast of their good health as a sign of God's favor since it was morality, not unmotivated blessing proved by physical well-being.[12]

Moral methodology is rooted in scripture where Mosaic law is redefined not as a literal mandate but as an inner, embodied attitude (Matt. 5:27–30). Internalization of morality emphasizes that morality expresses both physical and psychological, as well as social or relational, benefits of living a moral life.

3. Affective methodologies: Affective methodologies recognize the role of emotions and the mind in determining health. The historical Eastern Christian perspective is at home in today's modern psychology and mental health fields. Most psychological approaches acknowledge the connection between mental and physical illness, or the body–mind relationship.

Alexander of Tralles (c. 525–605 CE), an eminent physician in Eastern Christendom, presented the affective methodology. Alexander has been called history's "first clinical author on psychotherapy"[13] as he demonstrated an appreciation for the significance of the emotional states of his patients. In cases where the brain was afflicted and other methods of treatment failed, Alexander isolated his patient and forbid visitors whom the patient found "upsetting." In other instances, he affirmed religious amulets and other spiritual medallions valued by his patients. Alexander argued that the patient's belief in a remedy could promote health because the patient would believe he would be healed.[14] This phenomenon is, in part, recognized today as the placebo effect.

4. Experiential (mystical) methodologies: The experiential methodology approaches healing through direct spiritual encounter. Many forms of what is currently known as "faith healing" existed in Eastern Christendom. These were rooted in direct spiritual experience through prayer, dreams, meditation, and mystical contemplation. For the patristic tradition and Eastern

Orthodox theology, mystical awareness is a foundation of theology and a means of healing. For instance, "The Miracles of St. Photeine" describes a blind man named Abraamios who prayed to God "not to neglect him who was in mortal danger, but to show him the path whereby he should not be deprived of the light that is sweetest to all men." Abraamios experienced God in a dream in which St. Photeine instructs him to dig up her relics from a burial site in a remote cave. Abraamios gathers some villagers, excavates the relics, reveres them, and is cured of his blindness. It is noteworthy that the villagers do question the legitimacy of Abraamios's dream, but they follow him immediately to the uncharted cave.[15] This conveys the seriousness with which Byzantines viewed mystical experiences that may find expression in dreams, as precursors to healing, as well as a belief in direct encounters with God.

For Eastern Orthodox Christians, mystical experiences are a means by which anyone may personally encounter the divine. The experiential methodology derives directly from Orthodox Christian anthropology and affirms the spiritual nature of personhood.

In the Eastern Orthodox tradition, mystical experience is the foundation of theology and a requirement for descriptive theology. Miraculous encounters or apophatic (beyond the mental/rational) theology informs cataphatic (mental/rational) theological expression. Apophatic theology infers a *theophany* (God-appearance) or *theoptia* (God-vision)—an experience beyond description. While God cannot be known, he can be experienced. The mystical experience is the foundation for Eastern Christian theological discourse. Because of this mystical, experiential requirement, Eastern Christians accommodate dreams, visions, visitations, and miracles as normative mediums in theology and as part of the mystery of divine healing.

5. Ontological methodologies: The ontological methodology views healing as the manifestation of those qualities unique to human nature; it is based on the theological tenet that God created humanity in his image and according to his likeness (Gen. 1:26). Orthodox Christians understand this statement to mean that qualities of perfectibility are intrinsic to humans and enable humanity to become like God, achieving *theosis*, union with God. While human beings are not perfect, the potential for perfection (through participation in God's energy) is present, as Christ describes, "What is impossible with men is possible with God" (Luke 18:297). When the innate qualities of perfection are activated and manifested through God's grace, we express our true nature. Patristic literature delineates the important human qualities in depth. St. Basil (d. 379 CE), St. Gregory of Nyssa (d. c. 394 CE), St. John of Damascus (d. 749 CE), and St. Cyril of Jerusalem (d. 386 CE), among others, wrote extensively on the innate gifts (so-called theological anthropology) of humankind, which include (1) innocence and spontaneity,

(2) rational faculties, (3) the capacity for moral perfection, (4) creativity, (5) free will, (6) spirituality, and (7) love. The basis of health for this methodology is to manifest these qualities, thereby experiencing one's potentiality, God's image in oneself toward likeness of God.[16]

6. Connatural methodologies: Relational dependency is the basic need and ability to love others where human nature is "naturally" expressed in relationship with self, others, and God. The connatural (meaning "born together") approach holds that human relationships are crucial to health and well-being. Fulfilling and loving relationships with self, others, and God are critical connections that lead to physical, mental, and spiritual health. This idea draws heavily on Jesus's statement that the greatest commandment is "love the Lord your God with all your heart and with all your soul and with all your mind and with all your strength. The second is this: Love your neighbor as yourself. There is no commandment greater than these" (Mark 12:29–31). Christ essentially defines the measure of personhood as love, a connatural methodology toward health, which explains fulfillment for human nature.

Healing Practices in Orthodox Christianity

Healing is central to Orthodox Christian living. The faithful express a wide range of spiritual practices that have provided both comfort and results throughout history. These include prayer, meditation, miracles and saints, and sacraments.

Prayer

Prayer is a medium for direct access to God. Orthodox Christianity is a faith of worship and a highly developed liturgical life. The etymology of the word *liturgy* comes from the Greek, meaning "work of the people." The intention of prayer is neither a public display or event but an experience of connection of the gathered faithful. As Christ says, "When two or three gather in my name there, I am with them" (Matt. 18:20). Prayer is a primary means for healing. Orthodox Christians regularly pray to Christ as well as saints who serve as intercessors for healing. St. Paul counsels us "to pray without ceasing" (1 Thess. 5:17). Icons adorn Orthodox Christian churches and are preserved in Orthodox Christian homes as windows to heaven, affirming a central teaching of the faith that the Kingdom of God is here yet not fully manifested. Orthodox Christians and other faithful denominations affirm the miracles of body, mind, and soul as a result of prayer.[17] The faithful attest to miracles as a result of direct divine intervention through prayer.[18]

Meditation

Because corporate or communal experience is central to practice in East-ern Orthodox Christianity, a theological principle of "unity and diversity" characterizes Orthodox Christian worship. The faithful are not required to conform to a particular engagement with God. Therefore, when attending church service, one may observe that the participants express "unity" as a congregation in belief and "diversity" in their particular engagements with God. A priest may lead prayer, invoke the Holy Spirit, or incense icons and the faithful. Congregants may petition aloud, while others follow the liturgy; some stand, others kneel; some sing, others meditate on an icon, pray silently, or meditate on a single word, engaging in contact with God. Meditation is different from prayer in that it is focused attention on God and contempla-tion of a specific subject, word, or event.

Orthodoxy retains a tradition of meditation or contemplation that may also be conducted in silence. Meditation in Eastern Orthodoxy is a means for resetting oneself, emerging from a long-standing monastic tradition, refined by the desert fathers and following St. Anthony the Great (the father of monasticism) from the third century CE. The prayers of silence used the "language of the kingdom of heaven" described by St. Isaac the Syrian, from the seventh century, and support meditation as unceasing prayer (1 Thess. 5:17). In the 11th century, St. Symeon the New Theologian detailed the pro-cess of "prayer of the heart." St. Gregory Palamas clarified hesychasm (silence or quiet prayer) as a transformative experience from a mental practice draw-ing upon repetition of the Jesus Prayer ("Lord Jesus Christ, have mercy upon me, a sinner."), leading to an elevated, transformed state. While an ecstatic state may be a secondary result of hesychasm, it is not the goal. St. Gregory Palamas explained that such energies of God can be experienced as a func-tion of meditative (hesychastic) spirituality.[19]

Miracles and Saints

For Orthodox Christianity, the "true miracle" is the revelation and revolu-tion inaugurated by Jesus Christ: his birth, ministry, crucifixion, and resur-rection. Jesus Christ empties himself into the fallen world (in Greek, *perichoresis*, or "self-emptying"), the miracle of God's intervention through the birth of Jesus Christ. Moreover, Christ's crucifixion serves as testimony of his love for humankind, where death is miraculously overridden through his resurrection. The lesson of the resurrection miracle is that humankind may share in the true miracle by participating in Christ's love and life in Christ.

While all miracles or healings are recognized in Orthodoxy as extraordi-nary, supernatural events remain secondary. Instances where the lame, blind, or dead are healed are temporary; the afflicted ultimately succumb to natural ends. However, the miracle of the resurrection of Jesus provides knowledge of the power and truth that prevails to the end of time, through eternity. Through the resurrection miracle, Christ shows that the love he embodied rules over space and time but is subject to neither. Sergius Bulgakov observes that the New Testament provides a series of texts with a common theme: "The Resurrection of Christ was accomplished in that 'God has raised up (in Greek, *anestesen*) Jesus of Nazareth.'"[20]

The miracle of the resurrection confirms Christ's authority beyond the limits of the world. The healing events of the New Testament, as well as those available through faith healings today, so-called secondary miracles, serve to affirm Christ's authority and draw attention to him; yet the miracle culminating in Christ's love in the resurrection transforms people. This miracle demonstrates Christ's ontological power, inviting followers to participate in his life through prayer, holiness, and love.

Although Jesus performed miracles, he was not especially inviting of those who sought out miracles as proof of his ministry and significance. The Gospels tell us that the Pharisees remained unconvinced of Jesus's claims about himself after he cured a possessed man who was both blind and mute. Following this event, the Pharisees accused Jesus of driving out demons by the power of Satan. They said to him, "Teacher, we want to see a sign from you." When asked to prove that he was indeed the Messiah, Jesus referenced the prophet Jonah to foretell his crucifixion and resurrection. He said, "A wicked and adulterous generation asks for a sign! But none will be given it except the sign of the prophet Jonah. For as Jonah was three days and three nights in the belly of a huge fish, so the Son of Man will be three days and three nights in the heart of the earth. The men of Nineveh will stand up at the judgment with this generation and condemn it; for they repented at the preaching of Jonah, and now something greater than Jonah is here" (Matt. 12:38–41). According to Jesus, the true miracle is the resurrection.

Orthodox Christians affirm miracles of saints and miracle workers as occurrences that encourage and strengthen faith. While some saints were medical professionals or healers, healing of body, mind, or soul within this psychosomatic tradition is frequently the hallmark for most saints. Saints serve as intercessors because of their spiritual achievements and affirm eternal spiritual life. The faithful therefore understand the church as "militant" in physical life and "triumphant" in participation of the eternal spiritual reality. Thus the saints are available as intercessors and mediators and to assist the faithful, much as one individual may assist another.

In line with a holistic understanding of healing, Orthodox faithful embrace the numerous miracles of professionals who seek to remedy illness and death through science and various healing acts. Jerislav Pelikan explains that the Orthodox "rich doctrine of creation implied the sacredness of the secular and the holiness of the natural."[21] John Meyendorff clarifies that all these "are feats of only temporary relief." Such miracles originate in science or religion as they share common goals: "to improve the quality of human life, to show concern for human suffering, and to try to alleviate pain."[22] In the last analysis, all these efforts, both religious and scientific, are precursors to a healed and restored world.

Miracles awaken people from their spiritual stupor, where faithful and unfaithful alike fail to recognize God in nature. Miracles occur as testimonies of faith both today and in the early church as a means of affirming the Gospel. Throughout the history of the Orthodox church, the Eastern Roman and Byzantine Empire's atmosphere of holistic healing in *xenones* (medical hospitals usually attached to churches) and hospitals drew on both medical and spiritual resources for healing, collaborating with patients' initiatives concerning their spiritual healing.[23]

Alice-Mary Talbot details a span of approximately 1,000 years during which miraculous healings occurred in Byzantium whereby many of the same illnesses suffered today were cured through miraculous healings at saints' shrines and sacred springs; through contact with the coffins and relics of saints, miraculous artifacts, and miraculous healing events; and by living saints.[24] Today, Orthodox Christians continue to participate in these same vital mediums for miracles in addition to engaging in prayer and sacramental life.

Sacraments

The sacraments of the Orthodox faith use liturgical experiences to heal both physical and spiritual dimensions in an effort to transform sensorial experiences. Byzantine art seeks to go beyond images of realism and, through hyperbole, expresses a renewed life through Christ. For example, for sight, icons demonstrate large eyes, conveying the new, wider vision through life in Christ; elongated ears point toward heaven to hear Christ's message; for smell, incense invokes a heavenly scent; for hearing, spiritual music awakens awareness of a new sound and message; for taste, the faithful receive the body and blood of Christ, recapitulating Christ's feeding of the crowds who heard his message; for touch, the faithful are anointed with holy unction for healing.

There are numerous sacraments within Orthodox Christianity, though seven are commonly identified: baptism, confirmation, confession, communion, matrimony, unction, and priestly orders. Although a specific healing focus is not explicit in the sacraments, they are all inherently acts that empower the presence of God. In particular, communion, which occurs in the Divine Liturgy, is replete with blessings for healing, which St. Ignatius called "the medicine for immortality."[25] Similarly, confession, while not the therapy or process for spiritual guidance and counseling, provides forgiveness of sins, healing, and a new beginning.

The sacrament of holy unction is the most explicit sacrament of healing. Derived from scriptures (James 5:14–16), it is among the original services of Christianity for healing of body and soul:

> Is anyone among you sick? Let them call the elders of the church to pray over them and anoint them with oil in the name of the Lord. And the prayer offered in faith will make the sick person well; the Lord will raise them up. If they have sinned, they will be forgiven. Therefore, confess your sins to each other and pray for each other so that you may be healed. The prayer of a righteous person is powerful and effective.[26]

The express purpose of the sacrament is healing and forgiveness. In addition to participating in these acts of healing, the faithful also wear a cross or blessed cloth called *phylacton* (in Greek, "that which protects"), visit shrines of saints and the Holy Land, and display icons for sanctification. While Eastern Orthodox Christianity imparts healing blessings for the faithful, ultimately, healing energy is accessed most directly through the embodiment of love as directed by Christ (Matt. 22:37–40). Ultimately, the manifestation of healing is secured through exemplifying virtue, goodness, and holiness (Matt. 25:35).

References

1. SS Kosmas and Damian were called the "unmercenaries" as they did not accept money for their services. There are three physician brother saints named Kosmas and Damian in Orthodox Christianity: SS Kosmas and Damian of Cilicia (Arabia), SS Kosmas and Damian of Asia Minor, and SS Kosmas and Damian of Rome.

2. Chirban, J. T. (2010). Holistic healing in Byzantium: Historical perspectives on Byzantine healing. In J. T. Chirban (Ed.), *Holistic healing in Byzantium* (pp. 3–33). Brookline, MA: Holy Cross Orthodox Press.

3. Schroeder, R. B. (2010). Healing the body, saving the soul: Viewing Christ's healing ministry in Byzantium. In J. T. Chirban (Ed.), *Holistic healing in Byzantium*, pp. 253–280. Brookline, MA: Holy Cross Orthodox Press.

4. Eftychiades, A. (1983). *Eisagoge eis een Vyzantinen therapeutiken* (Introduction to Byzantine healing). Athens, Greece: Graphikes Teknes.

5. Constas, N. (2002). An apology for the cult of saints in cate antiquity: Eustratius Presbyter of Constantinople, on the state of souls after death. *Journal of Early Christian Studies, 10*(2), 267–285.

6. Chirban, J. T. (1986). Developmental stages in Eastern Orthodox Christianity. In K. Wilbur (Ed.), *Transformations of consciousness: Conventional and contemplative perspectives on development,* pp. 285–314. Boston, MA: Shambala.

7. Chirban, J. T. (2012). Orthodox Christianity and mental health. In A. Casiday (Ed.), *Orthodox Christian world* (pp. 547–567). Nashville, TN: Rutledge Hill Press.

8. Basil, Saint. (1955). St. Basil's letters. In P. Schaff & H. Ware (Trans.), *The Nicene and post-Nicene fathers* (Vol. 8). Grand Rapids, MI: Luthers.

9. Sonderkamp, J. (1984). Theophanes Nonnus: Medicine in the circle of Constantine Prophyrogenitus. *Dumbarton Oaks Papers, 38,* 29–42. Washington, DC: Symposium on Byzantine Medicine.

10. Talbot, A.-M. (1994). The miracles of St. Photeine. *A Journal of Critical Hagiography (Analecta Bolandia), 112*(1), 85–104. Brussels, Belgium: Societé des Bollandistes.

11. Seeman, T. E., Dubin, L. F., & Seeman, M. (2003). Religiosity/spirituality and health: A critical review of the evidence for biological pathways. *American Psychologist, 58*(1), 53–63.

12. Nutton, V. (1984). From Galen to Alexander: Aspects of medicine and medical practice in late antiquity. *Dumbarton Oaks Papers, 38,* 1–14. Washington, DC: Symposium on Byzantine Medicine.

13. Chirban, J. T. (2012). Orthodox Christianity and mental health. In A. Casiday (Ed.), *Orthodox Christian world* (pp. 547–567). Nashville, TN: Rutledge Hill Press.

14. Taton, R. (1964). *Ancient and medieval science from the beginnings to 1450* (A. J. Pomerans, Trans.). New York: Basic Books.

15. Talbot, A.-M. (1994). The miracles of St. Photeteine. *A Journal of Critical Hagiography (Analecta Bolandia), 112*(1), 85–104. Brussels, Belgium: Societé des Bollandistes.

16. Chirban, J. T. (2001). The path of growth and development in Eastern Orthodoxy. In J. T. Chirban (Ed.), *Sickness or sin? Spiritual discernment and differential diagnosis* (pp. 15–16). Brookline, MA: Holy Cross Orthodox Press.

17. NewsmaxHealth. (2015). Science proves the healing power of prayer. Retrieved on March 12, 2018, from http://www.newsmax.com/Health/Headline /prayer-health-faith-medicine/2015/03/31/id/635623/

18. Orthodox Christian Parenting. (2017). On miracles that God performs through icons. Retrieved on March 12, 2018, from https://orthodoxchristianparenting.wordpress.com/category/miracles/

19. Meyendoreff, J. (1974). *St. Gregory Palamas and Orthodox spirituality.* Yonkers, NY: St. Vladimir's Press.

20. Bulgakov, S. (2011). *Relics and miracles.* Grand Rapids, MI: William B. Eerdmans Publishing.

21. Pelikan, J. (2010). Foreword. In J. T. Chirban (Ed.), *Holistic healing in Byzantium* (p. xii). Brookline, MA: Holy Cross Press.

22. Meyendorff, J. (1991). Miracles—religious reflections. In J. T. Chirban (Ed.), *Healing* (p. 54). Brookline, MA: Holy Cross Press.

23. Miller, T. (2010). Byzantine hospitals and holistic medicine. In J. T. Chirban (Ed.), *Holistic healing in Byzantium* (pp. 73–85). Brookline, MA: Holy Cross Press.

24. Talbot, A.-M. (2010). Faith healing in Byzantium. In J. T. Chirban (Ed.), *Holistic healing in Byzantium* (pp. 151–172). Brookline, MA: Holy Cross Press.

25. New Advent. (n.d.). The epistle of Ignatius to the Ephesians. Retrieved on March 12, 2018, from http://www.newadvent.org/fathers/0104.htm

26. Papadeas, G. L. (Ed. and Trans.). (2007). *Greek Orthodox holy week and Easter services.* South Daytona, FL: Patmos Press.

CHAPTER THIRTEEN

The Effects of Religious and Spiritual Interventions on Pain

Amy Wachholtz and Christina E. Fitch

In the United States, over 30 percent of adults live with chronic pain. One-third of those individuals experience severe daily pain.[1] Overall, chronic pain results in an annual cost of between $560 and $635 billion from health-care costs and reduced productivity. This is greater than the costs of heart disease, cancer, and diabetes.[2] Individuals with chronic pain experience serious impacts on their quality of life, not only from the pain itself but also from the comorbidities that often accompany chronic pain, including depression, anxiety, and sleep disruption.[3]

Pain is a complex and multidimensional issue that affects (and is affected by) our biological, psychological, social, and religious/spiritual (R/S) health. Spirituality, in turn, is a complex domain that includes religious components and potentially a relationship with a higher power. For the purposes of this chapter, we will use Pargament's definition of religion as a search for significance in ways related to the sacred.[4] In contrast, spirituality is related to the integration and expression of that search.

Pain and spirituality have a two-way relationship. Pain can affect spiritual health, while at the same time, spiritual resources can exacerbate or ameliorate the pain experience. While spirituality used to be considered a passive form of coping, more recent research has identified that the use of religious and spiritual coping resources is actually an active and engaged form of pain management.

Individuals may use their religious and spiritual coping resources to manage their chronic pain condition. Styles of religious coping may vary based on cultural and religious factors as well as personality and situational factors. Usually individuals repeatedly rely on the same coping strategies over time. However, situational factors, such as experiencing a chronic pain condition, especially those that challenge an individual beyond his or her usual personal resources, may trigger the use of novel R/S coping strategies.

Models of Pain and Spirituality

There are a number of models of religious coping in relation to health. Most models for research and clinical practice focus on transreligious forms of R/S rather than examining individual religious groups. While this is not an attempt to diminish the uniqueness of individual religious groups, it is an attempt to identify universal mechanisms and outcomes that can be used to identify how R/S coping affects individuals regardless of specific religious orientation. While we will present the basic outlines of R/S and health models in this chapter, we recommend examining the source references for a fuller description of the individual models.

A universal model for R/S influence on health was presented by Park and colleagues to outline a general approach of researchers and may be useful for those who are otherwise unfamiliar with R/S approaches to health (see Figure 13.1).[5] This is a streamlined universal model from a more multifaceted model presented by Aldwin and colleagues that provides more specific pathways based primarily on U.S.-based research (see Figure 13.2).[6]

The most basic model of R/S influences on health, and perhaps the easiest to use in a clinical setting, is designating "positive" and "negative" R/S coping, where positive and negative forms of religious coping are related to empirically validated adaptive versus maladaptive cognition, affect, and behavior. Generally, positive forms include positive affect toward a higher power and feeling that one has a loving and supportive relationship with God. Positive forms are empirically associated with better mental, physical, spiritual, and existential outcomes, including reducing a patient's pain experiences and improving pain-related daily functioning. Positive spiritual

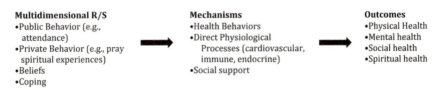

Figure 13.1   General Model R/S Influence on Health

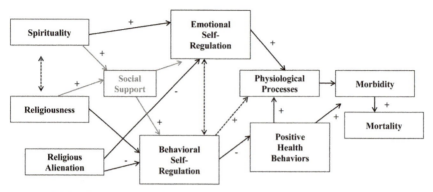

Figure 13.2 Pathways Model for R/S Influence on General Health from U.S.-Based Research

practices may assist with pain management by distracting, reducing stress, and providing social interaction and spiritual support. It might also regulate serotonin pathways to improve mood. In contrast, negative forms of coping include long-term negative emotions directed toward a higher power, including fear, anger, and feelings of abandonment with corresponding thoughts and behaviors associated with this negative affect. Negative R/S has been shown to specifically increase pain sensitivity and decrease pain tolerance. In general, negative forms of religious coping have strong evidence for increased morbidity and mortality among physically healthy and medically ill patients, even after controlling for mental health conditions such as depression and anxiety.[7]

A more extensive model that expands beyond the simple "good/bad" dichotomy was proposed by Pargament and colleagues.[8] In this model, there are four different R/S coping styles regarding the relationship with a higher power: deferring, collaborative, abandon/punish, and independent.[9] Deferring style is when the individual takes no personal responsibility for their health but defers all health decisions/activities to a higher power. Collaborative style is when the individual takes responsibility for the things they can control but uses R/S resources to support those efforts. These individuals tend to have the best multidimensional health outcomes. The independent style is when an individual does not include a higher power in their health approach due to no belief, but there is no emotional content in the lack of relationship. Abandon style is when there is no R/S involvement because the individual feels abandoned, punished, or angry with the higher power. Across multiple studies, the abandon group has shown the worst mental, physical, and spiritual health outcomes. This model and assessment tools based on this model have been validated in Jewish, Christian, Hindu, Buddhist, and Muslim populations. During the validation process, Pargament's

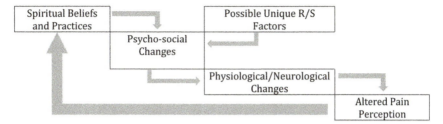

Figure 13.3   Psycho-Social-Physiological Pathways between R/S and Pain

team identified specific factors regarding religious groups, including unique benefits depending on religious group, level of religiosity, and type of stressful situation.

Another model that more explicitly explores the psycho-spiritual-physiological pathways and pain outcomes was proposed by Wachholtz, Pearce, and Koenig.[10] This model integrates the bio-psycho-social-spiritual model of health along with the gate/neuromatrix model of pain that identifies the role of psychological factors in exacerbating or ameliorating the pain experience.[11] This model proposes a feedback loop between R/S practices and pain perception in that individuals who are successful at using R/S resources to manage pain are more likely to continue to use their R/S resources to manage their pain. The coping pattern may cause alterations regarding their R/S beliefs, cognitions about efficacy, and their relationship with their higher power (see Figure 13.3).

A number of models are also beginning to include the concept of meaning making in their pain-coping models. Research has shown that existential meaning making, using R/S meaning making to identify a purpose, can create changes to the long-term pain experience.[12] Meaning making can reduce inflammation and decrease psychological stress in a way that aligns with the individual's world view using either explicitly R/S meaning making or potentially secular existential meaning making.

Existential distress includes the loss of a sense of self and loss of societal role. It is often used in R/S literature as a potential intersection between spiritual models and secular models of health, since spirituality is viewed as the sense of connectedness to other individuals and the Divine. Existential distress has not been empirically tested while embedded in a model of spirituality and pain. However, it has been included in some theoretical models, such as Dame Cecily Saunders's concept of total pain.[13] While not tested, there is theoretical validity to include existential distress in the model, since any form of distress is likely to increase inflammatory factors, increase likelihood of anxiety or depression, and increase the pain experience. Erik Erikson developed the psychosocial stages of development from infant to adulthood and indicated that distress can occur when the individual is out of step with their age-appropriate stage.[14] Since chronic pain may interfere with the largest stage (generativity vs. stagnation), and the age at which most chronic pain develops (40–65 years old) coincides, this may cause psycho-social-existential distress when pain interferes with the individual's ability to be a productive and caring individual in society.

There are differences among the models, but there is universal recognition that there are psychological, social, spiritual, and biological components that influence the experience of pain. Models are continuing to develop as empirical research provides more information on how various factors influence this relationship to inform research, clinical, and personal practice of pain management.

Historical/Cultural Perspectives

The differences between religion and spirituality and their impact on the experience of pain can sometimes be confounded by cultural beliefs and values. Within a religious tradition, there can be heterogeneous views of pain and its meaning; therefore, it would be a fallacy to draw expansive conclusions that those who ascribe to a certain religious tradition have the same perceptions of pain and meaning making. In light of this, we should practice cultural/spiritual humility rather than assume competence if we are aware of a trend among one spiritual group.[15] That being said, research has shown some trends within religious communities.

In general, religions attempt to rationalize suffering as a fundamental human experience and make meaning from this unavoidable situation. It makes sense that spirituality would be the element of the multifaceted human being that would grapple with this quandary as faith or a belief system helps people to "transcend suffering and to live with its mystery" (p. 84).[16]

An interesting and often overlooked piece of information is that more than 20 percent of Americans with chronic pain do not seek traditional medical care for their pain. This statistic is replicated in studies with homogenous ethnic demographics but has not been studied explicitly in more diverse cultural or ethnic populations. There is minimal empirical data in some religious subgroups, such as Muslims, compared to other groups, such as African American Christians and American Indians. Therefore, more targeted pain research on diverse ethnic and religious groups would help us understand if this statistic applies to all facets of the American populace.[17] Fundamentally, if one spiritual or ethnic subgroup uses fewer biomedical treatments for pain and focuses more on the holistic treatment of pain (biological, psychological, social, and spiritual aspects), this could greatly affect the pain experience.

Among some Muslim populations, there is a sense that if they feel more pain at the end of their life, this will result in less pain between death and burial.[18] Likewise, some practitioners of the Muslim faith feel that they benefit from increased faith as an effect of enduring suffering or that pain is a test of faith.[19] So, reflecting back on the models of spiritual coping, these would be examples of positive meaning making or collaborative coping.

A specific ethnic population in the United States that has a higher-than-average prevalence of chronic pain and pain-related issues is the American Indian (AI) people, according to 11 of 12 studies in a clinical review of AI populations.[20] In fact, pain is one of the most common reasons for which American Indians seek care. However, Western biomedicine may not be the only type of treatment they are exploring for their pain; many will also be seeking support from traditional health practices. The most common reason to seek traditional healing is for pain, such as arthritis, chronic abdominal pain, or chest pain. Traditional health practices are broad in scope and address the biopsychosocial and spiritual aspects of suffering from chronic pain. Some examples are "sweat lodge (ceremonial sauna), feasting (strengthening process), pipes (ceremonial herb and tobacco), and storytelling (nonhierarchical environment for verbal communication).[21]" Such methods are spiritual in nature in that they increase the feelings of connectedness within the community as well as with the sacred. Contact with a traditional healer came with a hope or expectation for improved spiritual well-being, balance, reassurance, and a sense of self-cleansing in addition to relief of pain.[21]

In a qualitative study of southwest American Indians about their experience of cancer pain, spiritual and cultural practices were innately integrated, even seen as a single entity. Spiritual practices were wide ranging, including community activities such as planting crops, cooking for or feeding the community, dancing, singing, and drumming. There was a sense of these spiritual or traditional AI practices setting the stage for healing, since spiritual healing requires both individual and community components. The interviewed AIs felt that they may have caused their cancer by straying from traditional ways, for example by not attending community ceremonial activities at an earlier stage in their life. AI patients often reported that traditional spiritual ceremonies were more important to their cancer treatment and addressing the cancer pain than chemotherapy, and as a result they chose to skip their chemotherapy in favor of a traditional practice. Participants reported that the emotional or spiritual pain experienced due to their cancer could not be described as separate from the physical suffering. This makes a clinical pain evaluation especially challenging to document with standard methods. Finally, there was not only a cultural sense that reporting pain was a weakness but also that cancer pain is inevitable and untreatable, so it is pointless to tell your doctor.[22]

In another study of American Indians, including Alaska Natives (ANs) and Aboriginal Canadian peoples, patterns of pain reporting and coping were investigated. One cultural trend that was determined through interview is what has been labeled "blocking," or an unwillingness to discuss pain at all. There is a sense that the health-care provider is expected to have enough empathy to perceive the patient's pain. If the patient discusses their pain, then it becomes real, so they tend not to report it, and therefore their trust in their provider is damaged if their expectations are not met.[20] In fact, AI/ANs were highly likely to rate their providers poorly and to have inadequate pain management. This may be due to a difference in conceptualization of pain. One example is a study of Pacific Northwest AI women, who have a broad understanding of health that includes mind, body, emotion, and spirit well-being, which is at odds with their providers' approach that the pain experience is comprised of physical pain that should be treated by pharmaceutics.[23]

Research among individuals in the African American (AA) community has identified themes in the relationship between spirituality and pain, although we recognize that there may be more diversity within a religious or ethnic group than between groups. Some AA Christian religious traditions encourage limiting complaints about pain due to a sense that this is part of the human condition in this world. There is also a sense that discussing pain may psychologically amplify it. Therefore, clinicians may find it difficult to complete a comprehensive pain assessment in this population if their patient is reticent to fully report pain.[24] The inevitable consequence is that underreported pain is never fully treated.

In a similar vein, AA Christian elders, not just by their ethnic culture but also by their spiritual tradition, may liken depression to "losing faith," and therefore they may not want to be diagnosed nor admit to a depressed mood.[25] As mentioned before, pain and mood are intimately connected. Since spiritual meaning making can affect access to care for mood, it is recommended that clinicians inquire as to a patient's spiritual and ethnic narrative if they resist referral to a mental health provider.[26]

Research has identified differences between AA and non-AA Christians in coping with cancer pain. African American Christians are more likely to use church attendance, faith community support, and personal prayer to cope with cancer pain than white or Hispanic Christians. AAs are also more likely to request chaplaincy support for pain compared to whites. While both AA and white individuals report a shared sense of blessing (gratitude to God), AAs spoke about feeling accompanied by God on their cancer-pain journey, finding meaning in the suffering, and transcending the self. Conversely, whites coped spiritually by not dwelling on their suffering (i.e., "giving it up to God").[27] Additional positive spiritual coping mechanisms for pain identified in this study were that AAs focus on their expectations of God's sovereignty, using humor, formal/informal support from spiritual communities, and role switching in using their suffering for good. White Christians in these focus groups used their expectations of God's omnipotence in gifting them more time to live and formal/informal support from their communities, but the latter was focused mainly on religious services rather than other interactions.

For Taiwanese advanced cancer patients, many of who experience pain, there is a cultural difference in assessment of spiritual suffering and meaning making. The general population self-reports as 87 percent non-Christian, so this is different from many studies based in the United States. A spiritual screening tool has been developed for use in Taiwan but may be applicable to other countries with similar spiritual demographics in Asia and to Americans of such descent. The six items assessed are fear of death, doubt about existence, doubt about life meaning and death, after-death uncertainty, unfulfilled wishes, and unwillingness to pass away because of concern for loved ones. In one study of advanced cancer patients, nonelderly patients (under 60 years old) reported more spiritual distress in the areas of fear of death, unfulfilled wishes, and an unwillingness to pass away due to concerns for loved ones. The nonelderly group also reported higher average levels of physical pain compared to elderly patients.[28]

While daily spiritual practices may differ among cultural groups, these practices have been shown to have an influence on the pain experience. Among Chinese Americans, daily spiritual experiences were not found to be related to pain. However, among Chinese American women, more frequent daily spiritual experiences were associated with a lower likelihood of using conventional pain medicine.[29]

Acknowledging that all patients have a unique cultural and personal background in relation to both spirituality and pain, patients should be routinely assessed for sources of strength and coping. Care providers should aim for awareness and humility in recognizing that culture, ethnicity, and religious/spiritual approaches alter the pain experience. Reviewing the scant research performed in certain subgroups, it is clear that assessing cultural expressivity of pain, sensitivities, and values is important to appropriate pain management.

Interventions

Epidemiological studies suggest that the use of spiritual and religious resources to help individuals cope or manage their health conditions is on the rise. And, the trend of increasing use of R/S resources cuts across the entire demographic spectrum: young–old, upper–lower socioeconomic status, and various insurance statuses and racial and ethnic groups.[30] The proliferation of correlational and characterization studies adds to the evidence that R/S is frequently used by patients struggling with chronic pain.

While there is a great deal of correlation and longitudinal cohort studies in pain and spirituality, there are fewer interventions that have been empirically validated in a wide range of chronic pain disorders. The research

Table 13.1   Types of R/S Interventions

R/S or Secular Interventions	Inherently R/S
Drumming	Religious/Spiritual Dance
Forgiveness	Prayer
Meditation	Religious Bibliotherapy
"Letting go"	Spiritual Exemplars
CBT or Psychotherapy	Religious Community Support
12 Step Programs	Spiritual Self-Examination
Community Service/Volunteering	Ritual
Mindfulness Practices	R/S Assessment

consistently suggests that interventions that increase positive R/S coping can result in reduced pain experience, improved pain tolerance, improved mood, and better quality of life.

A number of interventions can be used to manage chronic pain (see table 13.1). Some of these types of interventions are inherently R/S, while other interventions can be secular or can integrate R/S components to allow patients to access their previously developed R/S resources as part of the intervention.

Regardless of which R/S intervention is chosen, R/S interventions are most appropriate for individuals who have an existing, stable, and positive faith history. If R/S interventions are implemented in the absence of this faith history, for example, in a situation where the individual has negative affective content related to their spirituality, or in a situation that could be considered proselytizing, it is likely to cause significant emotional distress and worse physical outcomes.[31] In situations with negative affective content around religious and spiritual belief systems, it is strongly recommended that interventions only be used under the close supervision of a psychologist or chaplain trained in spiritual psychotherapy.

There is an ongoing discussion in the literature regarding whether mindfulness and other meditation techniques must inherently have a spiritual quality.[32] Since mindfulness practices have been an integral part of the Buddhist religious meditative tradition for millennia, and other meditation practices with spiritual intent have been developed and practiced by thousands of religious and ethnic cultures throughout history, some argue that meditation practices cannot be stripped of their R/S nature. Despite this ongoing controversy, there is a significant body of evidence supporting the use of meditation interventions to treat acute and chronic pain.[33,34]

In addition to meditation, spiritually integrated psychotherapy has been found to be extremely beneficial to patients with improvements across psychological, biological, social, and spiritual domains.[35] Spiritually integrated psychotherapy allows the patient to address comorbid mental health issues, such as depression, anxiety, self-identity, self-esteem, and changing social relationships that can exacerbate pain in addition to existential and spiritual issues. This often results in more positive outcomes than a single technique or approach (e.g., meditation only). A spiritually integrated psychotherapy approach may include common cognitive-behavior therapy techniques, such as challenging cognitive distortions and behavioral activation, but may also include spiritual bibliotherapy (i.e., reading religious texts), use of spiritual exemplars (e.g., Catholic saints, famous rabbis), or spiritual self-identity examination.[36] The use of these methods aids in cognitive-behavior therapy for those who are already steeped in R/S because the meaning making of challenges including pain is supported by the R/S world view. Psychotherapy approaches are more complex and more interactive than a meditation technique. Furthermore, since they are based in psychotherapy, and often include a therapist treatment manual or patient workbook, the intervention needs to be provided by a licensed mental health professional trained in working with spiritual issues. While there is significant support for this type of intervention for chronic pain, due to the lack of well-trained clinicians who can implement these types of therapies, they tend to be used less in medical settings than in meditation interventions, which are much easier to implement because they require less investment in the clinical workforce.

Cancer Pain

Oncologic pain is physical pain that stems from the original cancer site or metastases or results from the treatment of the cancer. Advanced disease-related pain (e.g., vertebral fracture due to bony metastasis), surgical or interventional pain, and side effects from chemotherapy or radiation are all included in the category of cancer pain. It has been well researched and is often separated in the research literature from other forms of pain due to its relatively well-understood physiological causes. Sources of oncologic pain can be either acute or chronic. In order to treat the pain and distress related to multiple forms of cancer pain, researchers have examined spiritual forms of meditation, such as mantram mindfulness and prayerful and Jyothi meditation. All these explicitly spiritual meditation forms were shown to effectively decrease pain, improve pain tolerance, and increase a sense of spiritual well-being among previously meditation-naïve patients. While spiritually explicit meditation interventions are now more widely accepted for use in medical care facilities among adults, there was initial uncertainty about using this technique with children due to concerns about inadvertent evangelizing and children's shorter attention spans. However, recent research has debunked these concerns and shows that the pediatric population can also benefit from the use of spiritual meditation to address oncologic pain.[37] Research has also supported the use of spiritually integrated psychotherapy for oncology patients, particularly in relationship to improving positive-affective forms of spirituality, which then affects both biological and psychological outcomes.[38,39] However, it should be noted that many (though not all) of the empirically validated spiritually based interventions in cancer are focused on breast-cancer patients, and future research would benefit from a broader range of cancer types and gender balance.

Among patients with advanced or life-limiting cancers, spirituality-based interventions can assist with pain, depression, and distress. While advanced cancer patients often show increasing pain and depression, spirituality-based psychotherapy has been shown to ameliorate the effect of increasing mental and physical health symptoms.[40] It should also be noted that there is a strong secondary benefit of effectively treating the distress of advanced cancer patients, in that it creates improvement in the primary caregiver's well-being.[41]

One of these interventions includes legacy therapy, a technique that often includes spiritual components but is not explicitly spiritual. It is often used in hospice settings to assist patients in identifying their lasting psycho-spiritual gifts to the world. In this form of life review, patients can reflect on lessons learned and emotionally close some chapters. The hope of legacy therapy is that the patient can find peace and healing in their relationships where there might be lingering psycho-social-spiritual pain that exacerbates the multidimensional pain experience. Some studies also provide patients with the means to advance that legacy through teaching others (e.g., patients, mental and physical health professionals) about their experiences to improve future experiences for others.[42] Depending on how legacy work is engaged, it may require oversight by a licensed mental health professional, since symptoms of depression, anxiety, and severe distress may become evident during the legacy work process.

Chronic Nononcologic Pain

Chronic musculoskeletal pain is a common problem among aging Americans. From low back pain to arthritis, 24 percent of Americans aged 50 or older experience moderate to severe chronic pain. Spirituality-based self-directed interventions to address chronic pain among older individuals have been moderately successful.[43] Empirical self-directed interventions have included techniques such as meditation, journaling with structured psycho-spiritual daily writing assignments, or videos with psycho-spiritual workbooks. While these interventions have shown moderate improvements in mental health and energy levels, the findings have been less exciting in terms of the pain findings.[44,45] However, these interventions may be very useful for patients who are homebound, those who do not have access to more robust interventions with a pain psychologist, or as a starting point prior to a more complete psycho-spiritual pain intervention program.

Manualized psycho-spiritual psychotherapy interventions, when delivered by a pain psychologist or other mental health professional, have been shown to have a strong, positive effect on pain and mental health across a wide variety of noncancer chronic pain conditions.[46] Psycho-spiritual interventions have been validated in genetic pain conditions (e.g., sickle cell),[47] acquired conditions with painful sequelae (e.g., HIV/AIDS),[36] and acute pain (e.g., emergency-room pain).[48]

Neurological conditions, such as migraine headaches, is one area with an extensive research literature supporting psycho-spiritual interventions to treat pain. Through a series of studies, spiritual forms of meditation have been shown to improve psycho-physiological responses to pain, reduce migraine headache frequency, and reduce the use of analgesic and rescue medications. Significant sustained positive results are achieved with 20 minutes daily practice for four weeks.[49] However, short-term results have been shown from a single 20-minute practice among previously meditation-naïve individuals.[48]

It should be noted that different types of professionals place different levels of importance on psycho-spiritual interventions to ease suffering and pain. These value differentiations are likely reflective of their unique training, which shifts individual perspectives. For example, when provided scenarios regarding different forms of patient suffering (a mixture of pain, existential distress, and depression) and asked about the most effective form of treatment, psychiatrists were more likely to estimate a high level of effectiveness for psychopharmacology. Psychologists, on the other hand, were more likely to rate supportive-expressive and meaning-centered approaches as highly effective, whereas nurses were most likely to rate comfortable environments and supportive-expressive approaches as most effective to address patient suffering. All disciplines rated explicitly religious approaches, psycho-education, and coping skills training as equally effective to treat multidimensional suffering.[50] While perception of effectiveness is not equal to actual effectiveness, it does speak to how health professionals approach patients' experience of suffering and what aspects they attend to in an effort to relieve suffering.

Conclusion

The experience of pain is a universal human eventuality; one cannot live without experiencing pain. However, physical pain is not the sole source of suffering. Pain due to psychological and social etiologies has been part of the dialogue in pain treatment models for some time. Less understood are the spiritual influences on pain.

The experience of pain can be mitigated or exacerbated by one's sense of spirituality. Both positive and negative forms of coping stem from spiritual interpretations of pain and the relationship a patient has with a higher power. Spiritual suffering, as one aspect of a person's experience of pain, can influence a person's total pain. Increasingly complex models of spiritual coping have developed as our understanding of the integrated person has progressed to connect coping mechanisms with the effects on the physiology of the patient.

Social-spiritual cultures and embedded spiritual beliefs have also been shown to influence pain response and meaning making. We have explored some research in different cultural and religious subgroups as well as different communities of sufferers (from chronic low back pain to cancer pain at end of life). The most salient conclusion of this brief review is that further research in more diverse populations is needed for further elucidation.

It has become clear that many suffering people rely on their spirituality or religious faith when coping with pain and that these R/S forms of coping affect health outcomes, including morbidity (e.g., depression) and mortality. Since empirically validated R/S interventions to assist with managing health conditions including pain are on the rise, all practitioners should understand how to integrate spiritual assessment and treatment plans. We look forward to future inroads into spiritually explicit interventions and psycho-spiritual support and hope that more practitioners will seek training in these influential modalities.

References

1. Johannes, C., Le, T., Zhou, X., Johnston, J., & Dworkin, R. (2010). The prevalence of chronic pain in United States adults: Results of an Internet-based survey. *Journal of Pain, 11*(11), 1230–1239. doi:10.1016/j.jpain.2010.07.002

2. Gaskin, D., & Richard, P. (2012). The economic costs of pain in the United States. *Journal of Pain, 13*(8), 715–724. doi:10.1016/j.jpain.2012.03.009

3. Baetz, M., & Bowen, R. (2008). Chronic pain and fatigue: Associations with religion and spirituality. *Pain Research and Management Journal, 13*(5), 383–388.

4. Pargament, K. I. (1997). *Psychology of religion and coping.* New York: Guilford Press.

5. Park, C. L., Masters, K. S., Salsman, J. M., Wachholtz, A., Clements, A. D., Salmoirago-Blotcher, E., . . . Wischenka, D. M. (2017). Advancing our understanding of religion and spirituality in the context of behavioral medicine. *Journal of Behavioral Medicine, 40*(1), 39–51. doi:10.1007/s10865-016-9755-5

6. Aldwin, C. M., Park, C. L., Jeong, Y.-J., & Nath, R. (2014). Differing pathways between religiousness, spirituality, and health: A self-regulation perspective. *Psychology of Religion and Spirituality, 6*(1), 9–21. http://dx.doi.org/10.1037/a0034416

7. Wachholtz, A. B., & Pearce, M. J. (2010). "Shaking the blues away": Energizing spiritual practices for the treatment of chronic pain. In T. Plante (Ed.), *Contemplative practices in action spirituality, meditation, and health* (pp. 205–224). Santa Barbara, CA: Praeger.

8. Pargament, K., Smith, B., Koenig, H., & Perez, L. (1998). Patterns of positive and negative religious coping with major life stressors. *Journal for the Scientific Study of Religion, 37*(4), 710–724.

9. Phillips, R. E., Pargament, K. I., Lynn, Q. K., & Crossley, C. D. (2004). Self-directing religious coping: A deistic god, abandoning god, or no god at all? *Journal for the Scientific Study of Religion, 43*(3), 409–418.

10. Wachholtz, A. B., Pearce, M. J., & Koenig, H. G. (2007). Exploring the relationship between spirituality, coping, and pain. *Journal of Behavioral Medicine, 30*(4), 311–318. doi:10.1007/s10865-007-9114-7

11. Melzack, R. (1999). From the gate to the neuromatrix. *Pain, 6*(S1), S121–S126. doi:10.1016/S0304-3959(99)00145-1

12. Dezutter, J., Luyckx, K., & Wachholtz, A. (2015). Meaning in life in chronic pain patients over time: Associations with pain experience and psychological well-being. *Journal of Behavioral Medicine, 38*(2), 384–396. doi:10.1007/s10865-014-9614-1

13. Saunders, C. (1964). Care of patients suffering from terminal illness at St. Joseph's Hospice. *Nursing Mirror, 14*, vii–x.

14. Erikson, E., & Erikson, J. (1998). *The life cycle completed.* New York: W. W. Norton.

15. Tervalon, M., & Murray-Garcia, J. (1998). Cultural humility versus cultural competence: A critical distinction in defining physician training outcomes in multicultural education. *Journal of Health Care for the Poor and Underserved, 9*(2), 117–125.

16. Heitman, E. (1992). The influence of values and culture in responses to suffering. In P. L. Stark & J. P. McGovern (Eds.), *The hidden dimension of illness: Human suffering* (pp. 81–103). New York: National League for Nursing Press.

17. Watkins, E., Wollan, P. C., Melton, L. J., & Yawn, B. P. (2006). Silent pain sufferers. *Mayo Clinic Proceedings, 81*, 167–171.

18. Firth, S. (2001). *Wider horizons: Care of the dying in a multicultural society.* London, England: National Council for Hospice and Specialist Palliative Care Services.

19. Reed, F. C. (2003). *Suffering and illness: Insights for caregivers.* Philadelphia, PA: F. A. Davis.

20. Jimenez, N., Garroutte, E., Kundu, A., Morales, L., & Buchwald, D. (2011). A review of the experience, epidemiology, and management of pain among American Indian, Alaska Native, and Aboriginal Canadian people. *American Pain Society, 12*(5), 511–522.

21. Greensky, C., Stapleton, M. A., Walsh, K., Gibbs, L., Abrahamson, J., Finnie, D. M., . . . Hooten, W. M. (2014). A qualitative study of traditional healing practices among American Indians with chronic pain. *Pain Medicine, 15*(10), 1795–1802.

22. Haozous, E. A., & Knobf, M. T. (2013). "All my tears were gone": Suffering and cancer pain in southwest American Indians. *Journal of Pain and Symptom Management, 45*(6), 1050–1060.

23. Strickland, C. J. (1999). The importance of qualitative research in addressing cultural relevance: Experiences from research with Pacific Northwest Indian women. *Health Care Women International, 20,* 517–525.

24. Meghani, S., & Houldin, A. (2007). The meanings of and attitudes about cancer pain among African Americans. *Oncology Nursing Forum, 34*(6), 1179–1186.

25. Wittink, C. (2009). Barriers to treatment and culturally endorsed coping strategies among depressed African-American older adults. *Aging and Mental Health, 14*(8), 971–983.

26. Morley, S., Eccleston, C., & Williams, A. (1999). Systematic review and meta-analysis of randomized controlled trials of cognitive behavior therapy and behavior therapy for chronic pain in adults, excluding headache. *Pain, 80,* 1–13.

27. Buck, H. G., & Meghani, S. H. (2012). Spiritual expressions of African American and Whites in cancer pain. *Journal of Holistic Nursing, 30*(2), 107–116.

28. Yang, C., Chiu, Y., Huang, C., Haung, Y., & Chuang, H. (2013). A comprehensive approach in hospice shared care in Taiwan: Nonelderly patients have more physical, psychosocial and spiritual suffering. *Kaohsiung Journal of Medical Sciences, 29,* 444–450.

29. Lo, G., Chen, J., Wasser, T., Portenoy, R., & Dhingra, L. (2016). Initial validation of the daily spiritual experiences scale in Chinese immigrants with cancer pain. *Journal of Pain and Symptom Management, 51*(2), 284–291.

30. Wachholtz, A., & Sambamoorthi, U. (2011). National trends in prayer use as a coping mechanism for health concerns: Changes from 2002 to 2007. *Psychology of Religion and Spirituality, 3*(2), 67–77. doi:10.1037/a0021598

31. Hollywell, C., & Walker, J. (2009). Private prayer as a suitable intervention for hospitalised patients: A critical review of the literature. *Journal of Clinical Nursing, 18*(5), 637–651.

32. Wachholtz, A., & Pargament, K. (2008). Migraines and meditation: Does spirituality matter? *Journal of Behavioral Medicine, 31*(4), 351–366. doi:10.1007/s10865-008-9159-2

33. Teixeira, M. E. (2008). Meditation as an intervention for chronic pain: An integrative review. *Holistic Nursing Practice, 4,* 225–234.

34. Hilton, L., Hempel, S., Ewing, B. A., Apaydin, E., Xenakis, L., Newberry, S., . . . Maglione, M. A. (2017). Mindfulness meditation for chronic pain: Systematic review and meta-analysis. *Annals of Behavioral Medicine, 51*(2), 199–213. doi:10.1007/s12160-016-9844-2

35. Pargament, K. (2011). *Spiritually integrated psychotherapy: Understanding and addressing the sacred.* New York: Guilford Press.

36. Pargament, K. I., McCarthy, S., Shah, P., Ano, G., Tarakeshwar, N., Wachholtz, A., . . . Duggan, J. (2004). Religion and HIV: A review of the literature and clinical implications. *Southern Medical Journal, 97*(12), 1201–1209.

37. Ahmed, M., Modak, S., & Sequeira, S. (2014). Acute pain relief after mantram meditation in children with neuroblastoma undergoing anti-GD2 monoclonal antibody therapy. *Journal of Pediatric Hematology/Oncology, 36*(2), 152–155. doi:10.1097/MPH.0000000000000024

38. Kaplar, M. E., Wachholtz, A. B., & O'Brien, W. H. (2004). The effect of religious and spiritual interventions on the biological, psychological, and spiritual outcomes of oncology patients. *Journal of Psychosocial Oncology, 22*(1), 39–49. doi:10.1300/J077v22n01_03

39. Jim, H. S. L., Pustejovsky, J. E., Park, C. L., Danhauer, S. C., Sherman, A. C., Fitchett, G., . . . Salsman, J. M. (2015). Religion, spirituality, and physical health in cancer patients: A meta-analysis. *Cancer, 121*(21), 3760–3768.

40. Cole, B. (2005). Spiritually-focused psychotherapy for people diagnosed with cancer: A pilot outcome study. *Mental Health, Religion, and Culture, 8,* 217–226.

41. Hebert, R. S., Arnold, R. M., & Schulz, R. (2007). Improving well-being in caregivers of terminally ill patients. Making the case for patient suffering as a focus for intervention research. *Journal of Pain and Symptom Management, 34*(5), 539–546.

42. Fitch, C., Tjia, J., Doering, A., Makowski, S., & Wachholtz, A. (2016). Impact of creating legacy teaching videos on well-being of advanced cancer patients. *Journal of Pain and Symptom Management, 51*(2), 456.

43. Lindberg, D. A. (2005). Integrative review of research related to meditation, spirituality, and the elderly. *Geriatric Nursing, 26*(6), 372–377.

44. Keefe, F., Affleck, G., Lefebvre, J., Underwood, L., Caldwell, D., Drew, J., . . . Pargament, K. (2001). Living with rheumatoid arthritis: The role of daily spirituality and daily religious and spiritual coping. *The Journal of Pain, 2*(2), 101–110.

45. McCauley, J., Haaz, S., Tarpley, M. J., Koenig, H. G., & Bartlett, S. J. (2011). A randomized controlled trial to assess effectiveness of a spiritually-based intervention to help chronically ill adults. *International Journal of Psychiatry in Medicine, 41*(1), 95–105.

46. Dedell, O., & Kaptan, G. (2013). Spirituality and religion in pain and pain management. *Health Psychology Research, 1,* e29.

47. O'Connell-Edwards, C., Edwards, C., Pearce, M., Wachholtz, A., Wood, M., Muhammad, M., . . . Robinson, E. (2009). Religious coping and pain associated with sickle cell disease: Exploration of a non-linear model. *Journal of African American Studies, 13*(1), 1–13. doi:10.1007/s12111-008-9063-4

48. Tonelli, M., & Wachholtz, A. (2014). Meditation-based treatment yielding immediate relief for meditation-naive migraineurs. *Pain Management Nursing, 15*(1), 36–40. doi:10.1016/j.pmn.2012.04.002

49. Wachholtz, A., Malone, C., & Pargament, K. (2017). Effect of different meditation types on migraine headache medication use. *Behavioral Medicine, 43*(1), 1–8. doi:10.1080/08964289.2015.1024601

50. Hirai, K., Morita, T., & Kashiwagi, T. (2016). Professionally perceived effectiveness of psychosocial interventions for existential suffering of terminally ill cancer patients. *Palliative Medicine, 17*(8), 688–694.

CHAPTER FOURTEEN

Spirituality-Based Interventions for Patients with Cancer

Andrea L. Canada and M. Elizabeth Lewis Hall

Upward of 90 percent of patients with cancer report using religion and/or spirituality to cope with the disease and its treatment. Although patients claim that religious and spiritual issues remain largely unaddressed in the health-care setting, there is evidence to suggest that individuals with cancer would be open to and benefit from such support. This chapter reviews selected efficacious randomized controlled clinical trials of spiritual and/or religious interventions in the oncology setting. Due to space limitations, the following four general types of interventions for patients with cancer are represented by two protocols each: (1) meaning-centered/meaning-making interventions, (2) mindfulness-based interventions, (3) moving meditation interventions, and (4) explicitly religious/spiritual interventions. Outcomes of interest include psychological, physical, and spiritual well-being. (Readers are referred elsewhere for more comprehensive reviews.[1-3]) The chapter concludes with a brief critique of the reviewed interventions and recommendations for future intervention development.

Meaning-Making Interventions

A sense of meaning and purpose is essential to quality of life in patients with terminal illnesses. Even when diagnosed in early stages, cancer can confront individuals with the threat of mortality. This threat is very real in advanced-stage cancer, often precipitating an existential crisis of meaning. Consequently, several programs have been developed to address meaning-making and existential concerns in cancer patients. Some of these are embedded in treatments that also contain supportive-expressive, cognitive-behavioral, or psychoeducational techniques. Given the variety of meaning-making treatments available, this section reviews two protocols that focus primarily on meaning making (in contrast to mixed approaches).

The most extensively studied effective meaning-making intervention in cancer patients is meaning-centered psychotherapy, developed by Breitbart and colleagues; this protocol has both individual (individual meaning-centered psychotherapy, IMCP[4]) and group (meaning-centered group psychotherapy, MCGP[5]) versions. The aim of this brief therapy is to help patients with advanced cancer sustain or enhance a sense of meaning, peace, and purpose in their lives by facilitating a reframe of their experience from that of dying to that of living meaningfully in the face of the threat of dying. The intervention is based on the work of Viktor Frankl and includes didactic teaching on the importance of meaning and the available sources of meaning, experiential group exercises and homework, and open-ended discussion for the purpose of emotional expression. The weekly intervention topics include an overview of concepts and sources of meaning; identity before and after cancer; life as a legacy that's been given (via the past), that is lived (via the present), and that is given (via the future); attitudes toward life's limitations; how lives have been created through family, work, community, and so on; connecting with life through love, beauty, and humor; and a final session inviting reflection and expression of hopes for the future.

The group version was tested on 172 patients with stage III or IV cancer, who were randomly assigned to eight weeks of either MCGP or a manualized supportive psychotherapy intervention (SGP).[6] The SGP focused on encouraging patients to share concerns about their cancer experience in a supportive context. A significant group × time interaction at two-month follow-up indicated stronger treatment effects for MCGP compared to SGP for quality of life, spiritual well-being, depression, hopelessness, desire for hastened death, and physical symptom distress. Examination of the change scores across time indicated moderate-to-strong treatment effects for all outcomes listed above in the MCGP sample but only improvements in depression for the SGP group. These results suggest that MCGP is more effective than a traditional group therapy approach and is particularly well suited to address symptoms of despair, such as desire for hastened death and hopelessness, in patients with advanced cancer.

Many patients cannot consistently attend group psychotherapy because of physical limitations, and this motivated the development of an individual version of the above program.[4] The individual protocol was tested on 120 patients with stage III or IV cancer, who were randomly assigned to receive

seven weeks of IMCP or therapeutic massage.[7] Therapeutic massage was chosen because it provides individualized time and attention and has demonstrated benefit with cancer patients by reducing anxiety, mood disturbance,
and physical symptom distress. Analyses at two-month follow-up indicated
greater treatment effects across time for IMCP compared to therapeutic massage in spiritual well-being, quality of life, and number of physical symptoms
endorsed and associated distress; little or no improvement on these variables
was evident in the therapeutic massage group. There were no significant differences between groups or across time in hopelessness, anxiety, or
depression.

The meaning-making intervention (MMi), developed by Virginia Lee and
colleagues,[8] considers the difficulty that is sometimes encountered in completing longer treatments with a cancer population. This intervention was
designed to be brief (one to four sessions) and tailored to the individual,
while allowing for flexibility in scheduling and the possibility of at-home
meetings. It has demonstrated efficacy in both early-stage and late-stage cancer. Finally, the authors note that this is the only existing intervention that
includes an exploration of existential meaning.

The MMi is an individualized and manualized treatment designed to
facilitate the search for meaning following a cancer diagnosis.[8] Its theory is
based on the recognition that meaning making is an important coping mechanism in the face of severe stress. The diagnosis of cancer is often profoundly
disorienting to patients, raising existential anxiety, and, consequently, this
intervention is intended to be administered shortly after diagnosis. The sessions are tailored to the patient's psychological and physical capacities and
focus on three tasks that are addressed sequentially. The first task addresses
situational meaning and involves reviewing the impact and meaning of the
cancer diagnosis with an emphasis on grieving losses. The second task
addresses global meaning and involves exploring past significant life events
and successful ways of coping, as related to the present cancer experience.
The focus of the third task is on existential meaning and involves discussing
life priorities and goal changes that give meaning to life in the context of
cancer-related limitations. MMi was first tested on 74 early-stage cancer
patients in a randomized controlled trial design.[8] Participants had been diagnosed with breast or colorectal cancer within the past six months and
were randomly assigned to receive MMi or to a usual care control group.
The results indicated significant improvement in the MMi group compared
to the control group on self-esteem, optimism, and self-efficacy following the
intervention.

In order to extend the findings of this study to late-stage cancer patients, a
pilot randomized controlled trial was also conducted with 24 recently diagnosed late-stage cancer patients.[9] Participants were randomly assigned to
receive MMi or to a wait-list control group. Given the small sample size of

this pilot study, only meaning was found to differ significantly between the groups, with medium effect sizes at one- and three-month follow-up. A statistical trend was also found for greater existential well-being and quality of life in MMi participants than in the control group three months after treatment. In addition, at follow-up, control-group patients were twice as likely to experience clinical levels of anxiety or depression when compared to the MMi group.

Mindfulness-Based Interventions

Mindfulness, rooted in Buddhist tradition, is the cultivation of a type of attention marked by nonjudgmental awareness, openness, curiosity, and acceptance of present internal and external experiences. Jon Kabat-Zinn westernized the concept and developed the mindfulness-based stress reduction (MBSR) program in 1979.[10] The standard MBSR curriculum is conducted in an eight-week structured group format, which includes weekly two-and-a-half-hour group sessions in addition to a six-hour daylong retreat. MBSR seeks to change the individual's relationship with stressful thoughts and events by decreasing emotional reactivity and enhancing cognitive appraisal.[11] Although initially developed for chronic pain, MBSR has demonstrated positive results in a variety of clinical and nonclinical populations, including cancer. This section reviews two more recent randomized controlled trials supporting the efficacy of MBSR on psychological and physical outcomes in patients with cancer.

Wurtzen and colleagues[12,13] conducted a population-based randomized controlled trial of MBSR (versus usual care) with 336 Danish women who had undergone surgery for breast cancer. Each MBSR participant underwent a precourse personal interview in which the concept of mindfulness and details of the intervention were introduced. The MBSR protocol involved eight weekly two-hour group sessions of training and included guided meditation, yoga, psychoeducation on stress and stress reactions, and group discussion on integrating mindfulness practices into daily life. A five-hour silent retreat was scheduled after the seventh week. Women were given a yoga mat for use at home and to bring to courses, four audio CDs of guided meditation, and a course folder containing didactic material on stress and yoga, homework assignments, and training logs. Sessions were led by one of three clinical psychologists trained in mindfulness. Larger reductions in the levels of depression and anxiety after 12-month follow-up were seen in the MBSR condition, with moderate-to-large effect sizes. In addition, greater decreases in anxiety and depression were seen among the intervention patients who were more heavily burdened by these symptoms at baseline. Furthermore, MBSR showed a significant effect on the burden of somatic symptoms post intervention and after six-month follow-up, but this finding was not maintained at 12-month follow-up. A statistically significant effect of MBSR on distress was found at all time points. Significant effects on mindfulness were seen after 6 and 12 months, but no significant effects were observed for spiritual well-being. The investigators claimed that theirs was the first randomized controlled trial with sufficient statistical power to provide evidence of a robust longer-term effect of MBSR on outcomes.

Targeting the specific psychological and behavioral concerns of young (i.e., diagnosed before or at 50 years of age) breast cancer survivors, Bower and colleagues[14] evaluated a mindfulness-based intervention to reduce stress, depression, and inflammatory activity in this population. A total of 71 survivors were randomly assigned to either the intervention condition or wait-list control. The intervention followed the mindful awareness practices (MAPs) program at UCLA[15] and was tailored for younger survivors by including information about prevention of cancer recurrence and maintenance of overall health. Survivors met weekly for six two-hour group sessions that included the presentation of materials on mindfulness, stress management, and the mind–body connection; actual practice of meditation and gentle movement exercises; and psychoeducation relevant to cancer survivors. Lectures, discussions, and group processes focused on solving problems concerning barriers to effective practice of mindfulness, working with difficult thoughts and emotions, managing pain, and cultivating loving kindness. Survivors were instructed to practice mindfulness techniques on a daily basis up to 20 minutes and to continue doing so once the intervention ended. The mindfulness intervention led to significant reductions in perceived stress, subjective sleep disturbance, hot flashes/night sweats, and fatigue from pre to post intervention relative to the wait-list control group. A similar trend was observed for depressive symptoms; however, the postintervention effects were not maintained at three-month follow-up. Postintervention mindfulness also led to significant reductions in proinflammatory gene expression and signaling, but there were no changes in plasma markers of inflammation. Strengths of this study are its focus on younger survivors, consideration of behavioral outcomes, and inclusion of biomarkers.

Moving-Meditation Interventions

Combining aspects of mindfulness with slow, purposeful movement, moving-meditation interventions for patients with cancer include such activities as yoga, tai chi, and qigong. These interventions are becoming increasingly popular and are offered to many patients through integrative medicine programs as part of comprehensive cancer care. Yoga, specifically hatha yoga, began as an ancient Hindu mind–body practice and consists of postures, relaxation, breathing exercises, and meditation. Qigong and tai chi, as practiced in the West, are similar forms of meditative-movement practices with origins in Buddhism. Generally, both involve specific movements of low intensity, focused breathing, relaxation, and consciousness. The goals of moving-meditation interventions are the achievement of optimal physical health and inner well-being.

Kiecolt-Glaser and colleagues[16] designed and implemented a randomized controlled three-month trial involving 200 breast cancer survivors assigned to either 12 weeks of 90-minute twice-per-week hatha yoga classes or a wait-list control. The authors provide a detailed description of the 24-session yoga protocol, which involves a number of gentle, slow-paced stretching and basic breathing exercises, in an appendix. A senior yoga teacher conducted the initial group, which was videotaped and used to train additional yoga-certified instructors. Survivors were strongly encouraged to practice the exercises at home and record total home plus class practice time in weekly logs. Survivors in the yoga condition demonstrated higher levels of vitality post treatment and at three-month follow-up and lower levels of fatigue at three-month follow-up. There were no differences between the yoga group and wait-list control group on level of depression. In addition, there were no differences between groups post treatment in markers of inflammation (i.e., cytokines: TNF-α, IL-6, and IL-1β); however, at three-month follow-up, the yoga participants had lower levels of all three cytokines (i.e., less inflammation). The authors conducted secondary analyses using yoga practice frequency as the independent variable; greater frequency of practice was associated with less fatigue, less depression, less inflammation, and greater vitality. Finally, the yoga group participants demonstrated improved sleep averaged across the two posttreatment follow-up time points. This study is noteworthy as it is the first published physical-activity trial to show significant changes in inflammation, a risk factor for chronic disease.

Larkey and colleagues[17] conducted a double-blind randomized controlled trial designed to examine the effects of a 12-week qigong/tai chi easy (QG/TCE) intervention versus a sham control on 87 breast cancer survivors' levels of fatigue, sleep quality, and depression. The QG/TCE protocol, designed to assist the participant in attaining deeply relaxed states, consists of a series of simple, repeated practices including body posture/movement, breath exercise, and meditation performed in synchrony. Sessions were one hour in length, home practice was encouraged, and participants maintained logs of time spent engaging in QG/TCE. (A detailed description of the intervention is provided in electronic supplementary material.) Decreases in fatigue scores were significantly greater for the QG/TCE intervention at both the postintervention and three-month follow-up compared to the sham control, demonstrating medium effect sizes. There were no statistically significant interactions on the measures of depression and sleep quality, suggesting no significant differences between the QG/TCE versus sham control groups' responses to the interventions across time. However, both depression and sleep quality showed significant improvements across time for both the QG/ TCE and control groups. The results of this study support the use of QG/ TCE for the treatment of fatigue in patients with cancer.

Explicitly Religious/Spiritual Interventions

Of the four categories of spirituality-based interventions for patients with cancer reviewed here, explicitly religious/spiritual interventions were the most challenging to identify in the literature. The two protocols to follow involve deliberate participant engagement with the sacred or transcendent.

Jafari and colleagues[18] conducted a randomized controlled trial of "spiritual therapy" with 65 Iranian Muslim women undergoing radiation therapy for breast cancer. Patients were randomized to either the intervention or to a control group. Participants in the control group received standard management, treatment, and education (about such topics as nutrition, physical activity, and radiation therapy). The intervention group received routine management/education and an additional six weekly sessions of spiritual therapy. Each session, led by experienced spiritual healers, was guided by a spiritual theme and concluded with a 20- to 30-minute guided relaxation and meditation exercise. Participants also received a 50-page manual and a CD containing written materials and the PowerPoint slides covered in each of the sessions. Each session lasted two to three hours and integrated didactic material, a question-and-answer period, sharing, reflecting, and relaxation and meditation practice. Themes guiding each of the six sessions included the following: (1) introducing the intervention and creating meaning out of the cancer experience; (2) learning relaxation and meditation skills; (3) giving to God those things under his control and viewing God as a supportive collaborator for things under the patient's control; (4) expressing grief and visualizing God as a witness to loss and pain; (5) enhancing relationships with self, others, and God, specifically expressing negative emotion toward God; and (6) praying to God for assistance. Results indicated that those who participated in spiritual therapy had better overall spiritual well-being (including higher levels of meaning, peace, and faith); better global quality of life (including improved physical, role, emotional, cognitive, and social functioning); and less fatigue, nausea/vomiting, pain, and sleep disturbance post intervention. Limitations of this study, acknowledged by the authors, included a small sample size, the lack of an "attention control group," and no follow-up program after six weeks to assess the long-term effects of the intervention.

In a study by Cole and colleagues,[19] 83 patients diagnosed with metastatic melanoma were randomly assigned either to a spirituality-focused meditation (SpM), a secular meditation (SM), or a usual-care control (UCC) condition. The investigators defined SpM as meditation based on explicitly spiritual content (e.g., images of God or Buddha) related to one's relationship to or identification with a transcendent being or force (e.g., God, Allah). This is in contrast to secular meditation that focuses on such things as breathing or imagery without reference to the transcendent. Intervention participants (in the SpM and SM conditions) met for five sessions over a four-month period. The intervention was delivered by two clinical psychologists. Each session began with approximately 40 minutes of assessing the participants' physical and emotional well-being and discussing the session theme. Session themes used in both conditions included maintaining quality of life, coping with loss of control, and self-care. In addition, in the SpM condition, the therapist in the first session asked participants about their religious history and current beliefs and practices, including the language and imagery they used to refer to the sacred, information that was integrated into the content of the sessions. In the last 20 minutes of each session, participants engaged in either relaxation exercises (SM), presented as a stress-management strategy, or in meditation (SpM), presented as a means to deepen spiritual resources for coping with cancer. The SM condition practiced standard relaxation protocols that focused on sensory modalities, such as deep breathing or autonomic muscle relaxation. The SpM participants engaged in spirituality-focused meditations related to the session theme. The following five meditations were presented: (1) time of meaning meditation, in which participants recalled a previous time of spiritual meaning to draw on that memory for support and meaning in coping with cancer; (2) healing-light meditation, in which participants envisioned a radiant light as representative of the sacred and a source of wholeness and completion and then reflected on one's spiritual hunger; (3) heart meditation, in which participants engaged in breathing exercises with a focus on the heart, fostering an awareness of and compassion toward one's needs; (4) letting-go meditation, in which participants were instructed to envision the presence of the sacred, ask "What do I most need to let go of?" and, as they let go, feel "bathed in a circle of white light, feeling acceptance, peace, and harmony"; and (5) spiritual-transformation meditation, in which participants envisioned the greatest source of compassion, breathed in that source, visualized it transforming them, and breathed that quality out into the world as a gift. Participants in both conditions were asked to practice the meditations or relaxation exercises daily at home and were provided written descriptions of the two simplest exercises and CD recordings of the others. Home meditation practice was also measured. Findings indicated that the SpM group reported significantly less depression and significantly greater positive affect than the UCC group across the four-month follow-up. The differences between the SpM and SM groups were not significant. Other quality-of-life outcomes as well as physical symptoms and mortality were not affected by the interventions. The strength of this study was designing a meditation intervention consistent with each participant's spiritual worldview instead of presenting a more "one size fits all" secular version. Although the authors report benefits of the SpM group compared with the UCC condition, no significant differences between SpM and SM participants were found. This finding may be more attributable to a lack of statistical power than an absence of treatment effects as only 20 (35.7 percent) participants attended all five intervention sessions. Replication of this protocol would be particularly informative.

Critique and Recommendations

In this chapter, we reviewed two protocols each of the four broad categories of spirituality-based interventions for patients with cancer. These included meaning-making, mindfulness, moving-meditation, and explicitly religious/spiritual protocols. Outcomes of interest included psychological (e.g., quality of life, depression, anxiety, hope/hopelessness, self-esteem, optimism, and self-efficacy) and physical (e.g., pain, fatigue, sleep quality, menopausal symptoms, nausea/vomiting, and markers of inflammation) well-being as well as spiritual well-being. Interventions varied from 1 to 12 sessions and were delivered by diverse personnel (e.g., psychologists, spiritual leaders, yoga instructors). Follow-up assessment times ranged from immediate to 12 months post intervention. Strengths of the studies include randomization with contrast control groups, relatively moderate-to-large sample sizes, and varied outcomes including biomarkers. For the most part, the spirituality-based interventions reviewed here have demonstrated efficacy in the oncology setting. However, we conclude the chapter with a general critique and recommendations for future interventions.

First, it is noteworthy that neither of the reviewed meaning-making interventions addressed religion or spirituality directly. As the most comprehensive meaning-making systems available, religions often figure prominently in meaning making, as does spirituality more generally. Consequently, even meaning-making systems that do not directly address religion are likely to draw explicitly on the religious resources of patients. Therefore, a significant limitation of the interventions reviewed here is their failure to explicitly recognize religion and spirituality as significant sources of meaning, and for many patients, the overall framework within which other sources of meaning are experienced. Failing to identify these as sources of meaning may implicitly communicate to participants that they should avoid spiritual or religious topics, depriving them of these important sources of meaning and unintentionally emphasizing secular sources of meaning. Given the centrality of religions in meaning making, it may also be useful to adapt the interventions for explicitly religious contexts, as interventions accommodated to specific religious groups often show enhanced effectiveness. For example, Pearce and colleagues[20] have developed religiously (i.e., Christianity,

Judaism, Islam, Buddhism, Hinduism) integrated CBT protocols for depression in the context of chronic illness.

Similar critiques of the mindfulness and moving-meditation interventions are offered. As the majority of patients with cancer use religion and/or spirituality to cope with the illness and its treatment, the fact that none of these interventions directly addressed or incorporated spiritual and/or religious content is potentially problematic. Secularized mindfulness practices and moving meditations may not be appealing to or as efficacious with religiously committed patients. Developing meditative interventions that include religious practices (e.g., contemplative/centering prayer, Lectio Divina, Muraqabah) or allowing each patient to select and practice meditations from his or her own religious tradition may increase their appeal.

Another concern is that, of the eight interventions reviewed here, only five reported effects on spiritual well-being. For many religiously committed individuals, spiritual well-being is the most important component of quality of life, especially in cases of advanced disease when physical and psychological resources may be depleted. Furthermore, all five protocols measuring spiritual well-being used the Functional Assessment of Chronic Illness Therapy—Spiritual Well-Being (FACIT-Sp) to do so. The FACIT-Sp has significant limitations as a measure of spiritual well-being.[21] Furthermore, one of the protocols[14] used only the meaning/purpose subscale, and another study[9] used only the meaning subscale of the FACIT-Sp, thereby excluding the contribution of faith to spiritual well-being. The FACIT-Sp is particularly limited as a measure of spiritual well-being when used without the faith subscale.[22]

In conclusion, we believe the efficacy of spirituality-based interventions for cancer patients, while currently strong, could be improved by the following: (1) as did the protocol by Cole and colleagues,[19] creating religiously accommodative protocols or, at least, explicitly informing patients that they may integrate their own religious beliefs and practices into the protocols and supporting such; (2) as did the protocol by Jafari and colleagues,[18] providing patients with the opportunity to express/process religious/spiritual struggle as appropriate in light of the fact that struggle has been implicated in health outcomes;[23] and (3) as also recommended in the review by Hulett and Armer,[1] meaningfully selecting and including standardized measures of the particular subdimensions of religiousness and spirituality that are relevant to the cancer experience and that are likely to be affected by spirituality-based interventions.

References

1. Hulett, J. M., & Armer, J. M. (2016). A systematic review of spiritually-based interventions and psychoneuroimmunological outcomes in breast cancer survivorship. *Integrative Cancer Therapies, 15*(4), 405–423.

2. Kruizinga, R., Hartog, I. D., Jacobs, M., Daams, J. G., Scherer-Rath, M., Schilderman, J. B. A. M., . . . Van Laarhoven, H. W. M. (2016). The effect of spiritual interventions addressing existential themes using a narrative approach on quality of life of cancer patients: A systematic review and meta-analysis. *Psycho-Oncology, 25,* 253–265.

3. Oh, P. J., & Kim, S. H. (2014). The effects of spiritual interventions in patients with cancer: A meta-analysis. *Oncology Nursing Forum, 41,* E290–E301.

4. Breitbart, W. S., & Poppito, S. R. (2014). *Individual meaning-centered psychotherapy for patients with advanced cancer: A treatment manual.* New York: Oxford University Press.

5. Breitbart, W. S., & Poppito, S. R. (2014). *Meaning-centered group psychotherapy for patients with advanced cancer: A treatment manual.* New York: Oxford University Press.

6. Breitbart, W., Rosenfeld, B., Pessin, H., Applebaum, A., Kulikowski, J., & Lichtenthal, W. G. (2015). Meaning-centered group psychotherapy: An effective intervention for improving psychological well-being in patients with advanced cancer. *Clinical Oncology, 7*(1), 749–754.

7. Breitbart, W. S., Poppito, S. R., Rosenfeld, B., Vickers, A. J., Li, Y., Abbey, J., . . . Cassileth, B. R. (2012). Pilot randomized controlled trial of individual meaning-centered psychotherapy for patients with advanced cancer. *Journal of Clinical Oncology, 30*(12), 1304–1309.

8. Lee, V., Cohen, S. R., Edgar, L., Laizner, A. M., & Gagnon, A. J. (2006). Meaning-making intervention during breast or colorectal cancer treatment improves self-esteem, optimism, and self-efficacy. *Social Science and Medicine, 62,* 3133–3145.

9. Henry, M., Cohen, S. R., Lee, V., Sauthier, P., Provencher, D., Drouin, P., . . . Mayo, N. (2010). The meaning-making intervention (MMi) appears to increase meaning in life in advanced ovarian cancer: A randomized controlled pilot study. *Psycho-Oncology, 19,* 1340–1347.

10. Kabat-Zinn, J., & Chapman-Waldrop, A. (1998). Compliance with an outpatient stress reduction program: Rates and predictors of program completion. *Journal of Behavioral Medicine, 11,* 333–352.

11. Teasdale, J. D., Segal, Z., & Williams, J. (1995). How does cognitive therapy prevent depressive relapse and why should attentional control (mindfulness) training help? *Behavior Research and Therapy, 33,* 25–39.

12. Würtzen, H., Dalton, S. O., Elsass, P., Sumbundu, A. D., Steding-Jensen, M., Karlsen, R. V., . . . Johansen, C. (2013). Mindfulness significantly reduces self-reported levels of anxiety and depression: Results of a randomized controlled trial among 336 Danish women treated for stage I–III breast cancer. *European Journal of Cancer, 49,* 1365–1373.

13. Würtzen, H., Dalton, S. O., Christensen, J., Andersen, K. K., Elsass, P., Flyger, H. L., . . . Johansen, C. (2015). Effect of mindfulness-based stress reduction on somatic symptoms, distress, mindfulness and spiritual wellbeing in women with breast cancer: Results of a randomized controlled trial. *Acta Oncologica, 54,* 712–719.

14. Bower, J. E., Crosswell, A. D., Stanton, A. L., Crespi, C. M., Winston, D., Arevalo, J., . . . Ganz, P. A. (2015). Mindfulness meditation for younger breast cancer survivors: A randomized controlled trial. *Cancer, 121*(8), 1231–1240.

15. UCLA Mindful Awareness Research Center. (n.d.) *Mindful Awareness Practices (MAPs).* Retrieved on March 12, 2018, from http://marc.ucla.edu/maps-classes

16. Kiecolt-Glaser, J. K., Bennett, J. M., Andridge, R., Peng, J., Shapiro, C. L., Malarkey, W. B., . . . Glaser, R. (2014). Yoga's impact on inflammation, mood, and fatigue in breast cancer survivors: A randomized controlled trial. *Journal of Clinical Oncology, 32,* 1040–1049.

17. Larkey, L. K., Roe, D. J., Weihs, K. L., Jahnke, R., Lopez, A. M., Rogers, C. E., & Guillen-Rodriguez, J. (2015). Randomized controlled trial of qigong/tai chi easy on cancer-related fatigue in breast cancer survivors. *Annals of Behavioral Medicine, 49*(2), 165–176.

18. Jafari, N., Farajzadegan, Z., Zamani, A., Bahrami, F., Emami, H., Loghmani, A., & Jafari, N. (2013). Spiritual therapy to improve the spiritual well-being of Iranian women with breast cancer: A randomized controlled trial. *Evidence-Based Complementary and Alternative Medicine: eCAM,* 353262.

19. Cole, B. S., Hopkins, C. M., Spiegel, J., Tisak, J., Agarwala, S., & Kirkwood, J. M. (2012). A randomised clinical trial of the effects of spiritually focused meditation for people with metastatic melanoma. *Mental Health, Religion & Culture, 15,* 161–174.

20. Pearce, M. J., Koenig, H. G., Robins, C. J., Nelson, B., Shaw, S. F., Cohen, H. J., & King, M. B. (2015). Religiously integrated cognitive behavioral therapy: A new method of treatment for major depression in patients with chronic medical illness. *Psychotherapy, 52*(1), 56–66.

21. Hall, D. E., Meador, K. G., & Koenig, H. G. (2008). Measuring religiousness in health research: Review and critique. *Journal of Religion and Health, 47*(2), 134–163.

22. Canada, A. L., Murphy, P. E., Fitchett, G., & Stein, K. (2016). Re-examining the contributions of faith, meaning and peace to quality of life: A report from the American Cancer Society's Studies of Cancer Survivors-II (SCS-II). *Annals of Behavioral Medicine, 50,* 79–86.

23. Pargament, K. I., Koenig, H. G., Tarakeshwar, N., & Hahn, J. (2001). Religious struggle as a predictor of mortality among medically ill elderly patients: A 2-year longitudinal study. *Archives of Internal Medicine, 161*(15), 1881–1885.

CHAPTER FIFTEEN

Religious and Spiritual Interventions for Obsessive-Compulsive Disorder

Timothy A. Sisemore

It is not uncommon to hear folks make light of obsessive-compulsive disorder (OCD) in public discourse. It is a humorous excuse for folks caught keeping the items on their plates from touching or organizing their desks in greater detail than others in the office. It becomes an almost cute quirk for many—one we can tease about because it is viewed as no big deal. While it may be true that most of us have an obsessive-compulsive tendency or two, that is not the same as having OCD. That is like saying if you've coughed a couple of times you know what chronic pneumonia is like. The dear folks who genuinely have OCD are disserved by such talk, and as clinicians, we want to understand OCD and offer the best treatment we can. I hope this chapter can facilitate better service to persons with OCD.

I will offer an overview of OCD, summarize the standard treatments, and then offer some suggestions on how these might be used more efficaciously for those who have religious or spiritual values or beliefs. A final section will focus on the uniquely religious component of many cases of OCD: scrupulosity.

A Brief Introduction to OCD

OCD may be the only psychological disorder with religious roots, as the scrupulous forms of OCD were noted in religious writings as early as the 16th century,[1] though Begley[2] argues one might go all the way back to the sixth century of the common era to a monk named John Climacus who noted the possibility of being compelled to think blasphemous thoughts by a nonself force, namely the devil.

Begley cites data from the National Institute of Mental Health estimating that 1.6 percent of Americans will develop OCD at some point during their lifetimes, a little lower than a broader range of studies cited by Worden and Tolin[3] that found a lifetime prevalence rate of 2 to 3 percent. The prevalence rate is only about half this in children,[2] often appearing at about 10 to 12 years of age or in emerging adulthood—though it is found in much younger children at times.

The *Diagnostic and Statistical Manual of Mental Disorders* (5th ed.)[4] criteria for OCD are fairly straightforward: the individual must have obsessions, compulsions, or both; these must be time consuming or clinically impairing; and the symptoms cannot be explained as the effects of a substance or other mental disorder. In this latest manual, OCD must be specified as to the person's insight into it, ranging from good insight that the obsessions are likely not true to insight absent, the person being convinced of the truth of the OCD beliefs.

The variety of types of obsessions and compulsions complicates the picture considerably. OCD is not just the stereotypical "handwashers." We will follow the concise summary of Worden and Tolin[3] to summarize the symptom patterns in OCD. Obsessions are recurrent intrusive thoughts that cause distress. There are numerous types of obsessions. Contamination fears include the fear of germs and the illness they may bring. Harming fears are persistent thoughts that the individual might harm him- or herself or someone else in some way (that might be violence, sexual assault, or even accidentally hitting someone while driving and not realizing it). Somatic obsessions include the discomfort of a person thinking his or her body or appearance is abnormal (and care must be taken to distinguish this from body dysmorphic disorder and hypochondriasis). Scrupulous obsessions are excessive concerns that one's thoughts or actions might be sinful or blasphemous—possibly leading to punishment from God. Similarly, some persons with OCD wrestle with "forbidden" thoughts, such as violent images or ego-dystonic sexual thoughts. OCD need not be limited to one of these. For example, among Muslims with OCD, religious purity is required for many religious rituals, and of the 10 forbidden things that make one impure, Muslims with OCD often obsess about being impure from urine, feces, blood, and alcoholic drinks.[5]

Worden and Tolin[3] note that persons who obsess often endorse maladaptive beliefs, such as an inflated sense of responsibility, a fusion between thought and action (to think it is to do it), a maladaptive belief that they can simply control the obsessive thoughts, difficulty tolerating uncertainty, perfectionistic thinking, and overestimation of threat.

Compulsions, then, are most often efforts to reduce the arousal and threat associated with the obsessions. These are tricky because they are negatively reinforcing. Washing one's hands when anxious about germs serves promptly to reduce the arousal—even though the relief is short-lived and leads to an increased urge to wash more later. As one of Begley's[2] interviewees cleverly noted, OCD is like poison ivy of the mind. If you scratch when it itches, it may feel good for a moment, but then it spreads and itches even more later.

Worden and Tolin[3] list several of the major categories of compulsions. Checking is repeatedly seeing if something was done, distrusting memory, and overestimating threat, and it sometimes flows from perfectionism. Excessive washing or cleaning has been touched on already. Repeating compulsions are redoing behaviors over and over (such as rereading or opening and closing doors). Mental rituals are particularly challenging as they are covert. These may be counting to oneself, saying prayers, or using certain phrases repetitively. Ordering or arranging involves manipulating things to fit rigid rules (alphabetizing books, etc.). Compulsions by proxy incorporate others into the rituals by asking them to decontaminate or reassure. I would add a danger for therapists is when clients try to pull providers into this by getting reassurance from well-meaning therapists.

All of this may climax in passive avoidance,[3] where persons with OCD alter their lifestyles, often to debilitating degrees, to avoid situations that might trigger OCD processes. It is often vital to address such avoidance in OCD treatment.

Treatment Approaches

As with many psychological problems, a variety of approaches to treatment have been tried through the years. Clearly, medication is an option in many cases, though sometimes it is given too quickly, prior to psychological treatments being given an adequate opportunity to work. Many times, it will be necessary to consider prescribing, but in general there may be wisdom in the therapist trying some of the following prior to referring for medication, unless the impairment to the person's functioning is severe and to the point that he or she cannot adequately function on a day-to-day basis.

We will focus on the psychotherapeutic options for OCD and then specifically on religious and spiritual adaptation. While many models of therapy start with a theory of OCD and built interventions from those, we will focus on the ones that have been shown to have the most empirical support.

Cognitive-behavioral therapy (CBT) is a broad group of approaches that incorporate aspects of thinking (cognition) and action (behavior). The preferred treatment methods for OCD flow from this genre. Cognitive therapy alone can be effective,[3,6] building generally on Beck's[7] model that sees negative emotions as flowing from maladaptive beliefs or appraisal. (This is specifically applied to OCD in chapter 11 of Clark and Beck[8] and in Purdon.[6]) It teaches those with OCD to identify those beliefs, change them, and test them against reality. With OCD, this may be altered to focus on patients giving up control of negative thoughts as disputing them may lead to an increase in the obsessions.[9] Despite the focus on exposure and response prevention (ERP), pure cognitive therapy may address important cognitive aspects missed in the behavioral focus of ERP and facilitate client buy-in to the challenges of ERP, a problem that is fairly common.[6]

Cognitive work is often foundational to working with persons with OCD, and pure cognitive therapy is being enhanced by approaches incorporating mindfulness. Persons dealing with OCD will vary in the degree to which they believe their obsessive thoughts and are best prepared for exposures (to be discussed shortly) by recognizing and distancing themselves from the "truth" value of the thoughts. Some mindfulness strategies are helpful in recognizing the obsessive thoughts,[10] learning to notice the thoughts without being caught up in the assumption that they are true. Defusing the thoughts from their meaning[11] can also facilitate this. For example, I often encourage clients to remember that "thoughts aren't facts." Even though some of the intense urges and uncomfortable feelings of OCD will persist, often good treatment begins by helping the sufferer disengage from believing in the intrusive thoughts.

Yet, the "gold standard" treatment for OCD lies on the behavioral side of CBT in exposure and response prevention, sometimes called exposure and ritual prevention. Rowa, Antony, and Swinson[12] cite data showing that up to 83 percent of persons receiving ERP improved to some extent, making it the treatment for OCD against which others are compared. ERP builds on notions of classical conditioning, with obsessions being associated with an elevated sense of distress that is then temporarily eased by compulsions. To break this pattern, one must resist the compulsions so as to eliminate the negative reinforcement pattern and then expose oneself to the discomfort until fear/arousal reduction occurs, thus loosening the association with the obsession.

Rowa and colleagues[12] provide a good summary of ERP that we will follow. As already mentioned, the initial challenge is to get clients to understand and agree to ERP. Given that the treatment involves them stepping in to things they likely have a long history of avoiding, assenting to this approach will require considerable courage and motivation. Explaining how it works and its long-term benefits will be important. We will return to this issue shortly.

Once the client is on board with ERP, an exposure hierarchy is developed based on a rating of subjective units of distress from 0 to 100. One then works with the client to see which situations cause what amount of distress. Rowa and colleagues'[12] illustration is a hierarchy for exposure to symmetry concerns where items range from a low of 35 for leaving a kitchen dish towel askew to 100 for client allowing his wife to put away clothes in any order. In contrast to some approaches that advocate flooding the person with exposure (though this still may be useful in some situations[13]), most practitioners take the client through gradual increases and allow the distress to subside in one setting before moving to more challenging ones.

Exposures come in several types.[14] In vivo exposure is likely the most powerful and involves actually being exposed in the real-world setting. If a person with OCD avoids hospitals for fear of getting sick, then going to visit a hospital is a great exposure. Sometimes one can create some exposure in the office, as I have done by having a person who avoids "germs" put his or her hand in a trash basket. Technology facilitates virtual exposures, though this involves expensive equipment. Finally, imaginal exposures are facing the feared situation in one's mind. These are vital when the obsessions are intrusive thoughts. I have offered some detailed suggestions on exposures elsewhere.[14]

Rowa and colleagues[12] suggest that exposures have a degree of control or predictability (contrasting with some who encourage surprises along the way). They also encourage more focus on the feared stimulus during exposure, rather than distraction. Here is another place mindfulness and acceptance skills may prove helpful.[10,11] There is some debate about the frequency and length of exposure sessions, yet the overall conclusion is that more often and more intense is better. Moreover, it is important that persons doing exposure be limited in escape behaviors (or compulsions) in the process, as these may interfere with fear reduction during the exposures.

Response prevention can be done by eliminating compulsive responses and safety behaviors (moving to places/situations where the anxiety lowers) or doing so gradually.[12] In outpatient treatment where the client will be responsible for most of the process, gradual is likely preferable. Helping the client in a sense undo the thing they avoid is helpful—such as keeping a "contaminated" rag on his or her person throughout the day. More moderately, the therapist can have the client "tease" the compulsion by defying it or doing something conflicting with it. Rowa and colleagues[12] rightly note that family members can help (or hurt) in the process. If family members are well informed and able to help with exposure in line with its principles, they can be helpful. Yet many persons with OCD draw reassurance and so much support from family members that their presence itself might be a safety source, thus undermining exposure.

Religious/Spiritual Enhancement of Exposure Therapy

The primary purpose of this book and thus this chapter is to show how religious and spiritual interventions can enhance treatment as used in harmony with the client's personal beliefs and values. The first way we will do this is to look at how a client's faith can be recruited to facilitate successful exposure therapy.

We noted above that while ERP has been shown to work, it is sometimes a challenge to get persons to do the hard work it involves. Yet, religion and spirituality have been thoroughly demonstrated to be used in coping with adversity in life. (See Sisemore's book[15] for an entire chapter summarizing this literature.) This raises the question, then, of how to incorporate faith in ERP.

Sometimes religious or spiritual beliefs can be helpful in the cognitive parts of therapy. In their more lucid moments, persons with OCD will sometimes acknowledge that in the eyes of a higher power or reality, their obsessive thoughts are not true. Affirming this may serve to strengthen them in not getting caught up in the doubts brought about when the intrusive thoughts are at work in them. For example, a Christian might affirm that God has changed his or her "heart" so that sin is odious. When OCD causes thoughts that one might harm another, this thought can be grounding.

But the greater role of spiritual and religious beliefs is seen in facilitating exposure therapy. Anecdotal evidence seems to support the idea that obsessive thoughts often undermine values and beliefs important to the individual. A person who loves children may fear being a pedophile, or a person whose health has been in jeopardy in the past may get caught up in concerns with getting sick. So it is that spiritual concerns may often lie close to the challenges presented by OCD.

It may be helpful to conceptualize ERP in the context of acceptance and commitment therapy[14] (ACT). Given the challenge of getting clients to do exposures that are difficult, ACT offers a couple of important constructs that may assist persons in doing exposures.

A short overview of ACT may be helpful here. ACT is a next-generation development in CBT that builds largely on recent developments in behaviorism and mindfulness approaches. (Hayes, Strosahl, and Wilson[11] is the standard articulation for ACT; a brief introduction is also available.[16]) ACT sees the key mental "virtue" to be psychological flexibility, leading to an acceptance of difficulties and suffering. More precisely, ACT sees the goal as a willingness to endure difficulties rather than avoid them. What would motivate a person to be willing to go through hardships? ACT says one will do so in the pursuit of what one values. While I might have slept in this morning, here I am at my office typing this chapter. Why? Because I value helping persons who suffer with OCD and hope my work this morning will serve this goal rather than my serving a lower value of extra sleep. ACT encourages one to know and pursue one's values in a way where one is willing to experience some discomfort in the process. I often illustrate this to clients with the famous workout mantra, "No pain, no gain." A person can't really hope to get in better physical shape without being willing to endure some sweat and soreness.

Now to connect the dots of ACT and OCD. If OCD tends to strike close to values, it often impairs the individual from living into what he or she values. If OCD attacks the individual with intrusive thoughts of being a pedophile, then the sufferer may avoid contact with his or her own child to avoid the intrusive thoughts and their accompanying anxiety.

Given that spiritual and religious values are highly salient for many persons, ACT would encourage recruiting these to help the person do exposures that offer hope for improvement of OCD. The careful therapist will have conducted a spiritual/religious assessment (see Pargament and Krumrei[17] for a good introduction to this process), and therefore be aware of the religious or spiritual values of the client and have obtained informed consent to incorporate these into treatment.

There are numerous religious principles and stories that may inspire the individual to do exposures across a variety of religious and spiritual traditions. A Muslim psychologist who works with OCD in Tehran uses the story of Abraham being ready to sacrifice Ishmael as he prepares his clients for exposure.[18] The Judeo-Christian version of the story is applied to Abraham's other son, Isaac, in Genesis 22 of the Bible, but in either case the point of the story is Abraham is asked to prove his faith in God as his ultimate value and is challenged to sacrifice his beloved son—another great personal value, yet subordinate to his faith in God. God allows Abraham to walk up to the edge of following through with this unthinkable act but then provides an alternate sacrifice and spares the son. Similarly, persons with OCD value the relief of avoidance but may mobilize their faith to do the hard work of exposure.

For Christians, one helpful verse from the Bible is Hebrews 12:2, where Jesus is offered as a model. The text observes that Jesus endured the suffering of the cross for the joy that was set before him. He went through suffering for the joy of fulfilling his spiritual mission, and so the person with OCD may live into his or her faith for the joy of overcoming the false intrusive thoughts of OCD.

Mojtaba Dalir[18] also enlists the wisdom of Imam Ali (A.S.), who stated that when one feels afraid or nervous to do a thing, then one should do it because the real harm you receive is less powerful than the expectation and fear. Here is religious authority for the notion of how avoidance is more damaging than facing the discomfort of obsessive thoughts and avoiding the compulsions that ease them. This would be helpful, for instance, with a person who does not go to work because he or she fears driving lest they unknowingly hit a person while driving.

An example of a spiritual value not associated with religion might be a oneness with and value of nature. Even here the value can be helpful. For example, a person with this value who fears germs might draw from this value to see the wastefulness of water in long showers and frequent handwashing.

Persons with religious and spiritual values are often wrapped into the meaning of life,[19] offering other strategies for combatting OCD. For example, many religious views value family, and, if we return to the fear of pedophilia as an example, one might encourage a client who sees his or her role as parent as sacred to step into interaction and even touch with his or her children as acting on this value in contrast to avoiding it to avoid the suffering of OCD feelings and thoughts. Similarly, a person whose contamination fears might keep him or her out of public might have religious values of visiting the sick or helping the poor that could add incentive to exposures. You may have the idea at this point.

In sum, particularly in the context of ACT, religious and spiritual beliefs and values serve as goals for life and thus increase willingness to step into contexts that OCD may lead clients to avoid. In so doing, exposure therapy can be enhanced. (Abramowitz, Deacon, and Whiteside[20] provide an excellent summary of exposure therapy for those who wish to know more.)

Religious and Spiritual Values in Scrupulosity

Finally, a few comments on an ancient variety of OCD: scrupulosity. As noted, this type of obsession may be the earliest form of the disorder noted in history. OCD often has a penchant for precision, and nowhere would precision or exactness be as important as in obeying God or following one's moral compass. It is one thing, though, to try to obey religious commands of not killing or stealing; it is another when scrupulosity gets involved to cause worry and guilt over having broken rules in the strictest, most literal sense. OCD can lead persons to see wrongdoing or moral failure in the smallest deed. Ciarrocchi simply defines scrupulosity as "seeing sin where there is none" (p. 5).[21] In an effort to do right by God, persons with scrupulous OCD can get completely bogged down in the fear that they did some trivial thing wrong. They may also fear they have blasphemed God in some way, or feel they are condemned by making a promise to God and not keeping it, or may believe they are hell-bound because they have not done the proper deeds or said the proper word to receive salvation. Such thinking does not limit itself to Christianity but can be found in other religions (hence my connection to Dr. Dalir in Tehran, who treats OCD in Muslims) or even to some who are not religious but obsess about violating some sense of moral precision (breaking an honor code, plagiarizing when writing, wronging someone by not saying just the right thing).

Several things about scrupulosity can create unique problems, and religious/spiritual interventions must be undertaken with care considering that. First, often the compulsion that accompanies scrupulous obsessions is confession and/or reassurance seeking. Persons with OCD who believe they have sinned may confess repetitively in prayer to God but also to religious leaders, persons close to them, or to "victims" who were never victimized. The therapist may also be used as a confessor as the client seeks reassurance from the provider that he or she has not sinned. Confession may be especially tricky for persons from religious traditions that formalize confession, such as the Roman Catholic Church. Santa[1] offers a helpful discussion and ends up encouraging the scrupulous person to have a regular confessor who may help tease out obsessions from actual sins.

Instead of confession, the person with scrupulous OCD may seek out reassurance that what he or she thinks or did is not a sin. This, too, serves to decrease the anxious arousal caused by the religious obsession and is a place where many well-meaning therapists may inadvertently be drawn in. If response prevention is part of effective treatment, it is vital that the therapist not reinforce the response of seeking reassurance. Rather, the therapist will want to work with the client to help other persons in his or her life not to facilitate this type of avoidance. Many therapists will benefit from insight from religious or spiritual leaders in the person's tradition to better understand how such scrupulous thoughts are managed in a particular type of faith. However, it may also be important to get permission from clients to coordinate care with their religious leaders or advisors so that care is harmonized and so these leaders understand how OCD works and why reassurance may actually hinder improvement.

Persons with scrupulous OCD may also develop patterns of avoiding religious triggers and contexts that stir OCD thoughts and feelings. Attending a religious service may create anxiety, as might praying or reading a sacred text. Such avoidance not only empowers the OCD by interfering more with normal life, but it may also undermine religious practices that support the faith that OCD is exploiting in scrupulosity. There are helpful resources in religion that can be mustered to help individuals cope (see, for example, Pargament[22]), and avoiding these may not only exacerbate OCD but also deprive the person of spiritual strength and community to stand against it.

In working directly with the scrupulous client, it may be helpful to clarify from the client's perspective the proper understanding of religious beliefs and develop a rationale that makes as clear as possible what might be "sin" and what likely is not. Persons with OCD often want more precision on this than is possible, but it can be helpful to define a basic rationale for distinguishing these. For instance, with a Christian client, one might say that the believer's sins are forgiven objectively in Christ's death on the cross, using this as a reason to give thanks when doubts and intrusive thoughts show up. Beyond that, the ACT approach to acceptance will discourage debating the thoughts and seek simply to identify them as OCD thoughts and remind oneself that "thoughts aren't facts," as noted earlier.

This sets up the challenge of imaginal exposure to the intrusive thoughts about possibly having done something wrong. Again drawing on Christian imagery, the story of Peter walking on water toward Jesus may be a good metaphor. When Peter looked at Jesus, he walked on water, but when he looked at the storm and the danger, he began to sink. Helping the person see the sacred as a resource of comfort and stability provides a powerful support for being willing not to argue with the scrupulous thought but sit with it while considering the higher religious value and truth. This is further enhanced by helping the client see how the scrupulous thoughts do more to hinder than help the life of faith and spirituality.

This approach can also be helpful in encouraging exposures to the avoided religious or spiritual settings. For example, wanting to obey the clearer command of God to pray or read scripture can motivate one to expose oneself to avoided stimuli while trying not to provoke worries about more minor "sins." All three of the major monotheisms value Abraham as a spiritual forebear, so the story of God calling him to leave his home and family and follow God without knowing where he was going can be helpful. This illustrates that faith involves acting on uncertainty and stepping into anxieties in service of the greater goal of following and obeying God. This is a critical principle to call to bear in dealing with many religious scruples.

Much more might be said to provide details on religious and spiritual interventions in OCD, but I hope this introduction makes the reader more understanding of OCD and particularly its religious and spiritual dimensions. I also hope it stimulates thoughts on working within the spiritual values of clients to promote change and progress against this persistent and insidious disorder.

References

1. Santa, T. M. (2007). *Understanding scrupulosity: Questions, helps, and encouragements.* Liguori, MO: Liguori/Triumph.

2. Begley, S. (2017). *Can't just stop.* New York: Simon & Schuster.

3. Worden, B., & Tolin, D. F. (2014). Obsessive-compulsive disorder in adults. In E. A. Storch & D. McKay (Eds.), *Obsessive-compulsive disorder and its*

spectrum: A life-span approach (pp. 13–35). Washington, DC: American Psychological Association.

4. American Psychiatric Association. (2013). *Diagnostic and statistical manual of mental disorders* (5th ed.). Washington, DC: Author.

5. M. Dalir, personal communication, August 30, 2017.

6. Purdon, C. (2007). Cognitive therapy for obsessive-compulsive disorder. In M. M. Antony, C. Purdon, & L. J. Summerfelt (Eds.), *Psychological treatment of obsessive-compulsive disorder: Fundamentals and beyond* (pp. 111–145). Washington, DC: American Psychological Association.

7. Beck, A. T. (1976). *Cognitive therapy of the emotional disorders.* New York: International Universities Press.

8. Clark, D. A., & Beck, A. T. (2010). *Cognitive therapy of anxiety disorders: Science and practice.* New York: Guilford Press.

9. Salkovskis, P. M. (1985). Obsessional-compulsive problems: A cognitive-behavioural analysis. *Behaviour Research and Therapy, 23,* 571–583. doi:10.1016/0005-7967(85)90105-6

10. Hershfield, J., & Corboy, T. (2013). *The mindfulness workbook for OCD: A guide to overcoming obsessions and compulsions using mindfulness and cognitive behavioral therapy.* Oakland, CA: New Harbinger.

11. Hayes, S. C., Strosahl, K. D, & Wilson, K. G. (2012). *Acceptance and commitment therapy: The process and practice of mindful change* (2nd ed.). New York: Guilford Press.

12. Rowa, K., Antony, M. M., & Swinson, R. P. (2007). Exposure and response prevention. In M. M. Antony, C. Purdon, & L. J. Summerfelt (Eds.), *Psychological treatment of obsessive-compulsive disorder: Fundamentals and beyond* (pp. 79–109). Washington, DC: American Psychological Association.

13. Fonenelle, L., Soares, I. D., Marques, C., Rangé, B., Mendlowicz, M. V., & Versiani, M. (2000). Sudden remission of obsessive-compulsive disorder by involuntary, massive exposure. *Canadian Journal of Psychiatry, 45,* 666–667.

14. Sisemore, T. A. (2012). *The clinician's guide to exposure therapies for anxiety spectrum disorders: Integrating techniques and applications for CBT, DBT, and ACT.* Oakland, CA: New Harbinger.

15. Sisemore, T. A. (2016). *The psychology of religion and spirituality: From the inside out.* New York: John Wiley & Sons.

16. Sisemore, T. A. (2017, January). I'm not broken, just stuck. *Counseling Today, 59*(7), 50–55.

17. Pargament, K. I., & Krumrei, E. J. (2009). Clinical assessment of clients' spirituality. In J. E. Aten & M. M. Leach (Eds.), *Spirituality and the therapeutic process: A comprehensive resource from intake to termination* (pp. 93–119). Washington, DC: American Psychological Association.

18. M. Dalir, personal communication, August 18, 2017.

19. Park, C. L. (2010). Making sense of the meaning literature: An integrative review of meaning making and its effects on adjustment to stressful life events. *Psychological Bulletin, 136,* 257–301. doi:10.1037/a0018301

20. Abramowitz, J. S., Deacon, B. J., & Whiteside, S. P. H. (2011). *Exposure therapy for anxiety: Principles and practice.* New York: Guilford Press.

21. Ciarrocchi, J. W. (1995). *The doubting disease: Help for scrupulosity and religious compulsions.* Mahwah, NJ: Paulist Press.

22. Pargament, K. I. (2007). *Spiritually integrated psychotherapy: Understanding and the sacred.* New York: Guilford Press.

CHAPTER SIXTEEN

Spiritual Practices and Interventions in Recovery from Addictions: Implementing Focused Treatment and Growth Strategies in Psychotherapy

Len Sperry and George Stoupas

Introduction: Addiction and Spirituality

In his 1961 letter to Bill Wilson, the cofounder of Alcoholics Anonymous, Carl Jung summarized the relationship between substance abuse and spirituality in the Latin motto *spiritus contra spiritum*: spirituality (*spiritus*) defends against the spirits (*spiritum*)—a common term for alcohol.[1] Spirituality has, in fact, been a core component of treatment in addictions.

This chapter presents some common and empirically supported spiritual interventions for addiction, including mindfulness, Twelve-Step Facilitation (TSF), and prayer. The chapter also addresses practical considerations for clinicians, such as when to introduce the subject of spirituality to clients, how to gauge their receptiveness, and how to use spirituality-based assessments. Finally, the chapter will end with an in-depth case study that illustrates these. First, we offer a brief history and rationale for the use spiritual interventions in the psychotherapeutic treatment of addictions.

Addiction is often referred to as a "spiritual illness." More than perhaps any other mental health condition, spiritual interventions for the treatment of substance-use disorders are both common and expected. In a recent survey, 74 percent of addiction treatment facilities reported using some form of spirituality-based intervention.[2] The significance of spirituality is supported by major organizations in the addictions field. The Substance Abuse and Mental Health Services Administration explicitly mentions spirituality in its *Eight Dimensions of Wellness*, noting the importance of "purpose and meaning in life."[3] Addressing spiritual issues is also included in the TAP 21 Addiction Counseling Competencies, the list of knowledge and tasks central to this field.[4]

The use of religion and spirituality as a means to combat addiction extends far back into the history of the United States. Long before Jung's letter to Bill Wilson, there existed a common belief that the solution to substance abuse was to be found in spiritual transformation. William James's *The Varieties of Religious Experience* lectures explored the role of religious conversion in the treatment of alcoholism, concluding that the only cure for "dipsomania" (alcoholism) is "religiomania."[5] This idea would be later advanced by Bill Wilson in the development of the Alcoholics Anonymous program in the 1930s and beyond. At present, there are a myriad of religious and spiritual practices found in addiction treatment, from traditional 12-step programs to Native American sweat lodge ceremonies.

As Miller[6] notes, spirituality can be seen as taboo for many clinicians, who may feel uncomfortable asking clients about their beliefs and practices—much less actively working to change them. Despite misgivings, however, the use of spiritual interventions in the treatment of addictions is well supported by research. Studies have demonstrated that religious involvement predicts lower risk for the development of substance-use disorders as well as for relapse.[7,8] Recovery from addiction is also associated with changes in a person's sense of spirituality. Sussman and colleagues[9] identify many possible reasons behind this association, including the development of personal morality, being of service to others, strengthening cognitive functioning, building social support, providing adaptive coping skills, and even the placebo effect. Most likely, the factors responsible for change depend on the individual and the specific spiritual intervention used.

Mindfulness

Mindfulness-based interventions (MBI) have become increasingly popular in the past two decades, with specific treatments now in place for problems ranging from depression to pain management. Sperry describes mindfulness as "a spiritual intervention separate from the formal practice of meditation . . . about being fully aware and attentive to the full range of experiences that exist here and now, moment to moment . . . [permitting] an individual to experience things directly and immediately, seeing for oneself what is present and true" (p. 210).[10] While mindfulness has roots in Buddhism, it can also be found in Christianity, Judaism, Islam, and other religious traditions. Jon Kabat-Zinn is commonly credited as the first person to systematically translate this spiritual practice into Western clinical practice with his mindfulness-based stress reduction. His definition of mindfulness, "paying attention in a particular way: on purpose, in the present moment, and non-judgmentally,"[11] casts mindfulness in cognitive terms devoid of its religious and spiritual origins, which may make it more palatable to secular individuals in the health-care community. While not without ethical concerns,[12] the use of mindfulness-based interventions is common and supported by research.

Mindfulness and Addiction

Addiction can be conceptualized as a drive toward wholeness that never materializes. The pain of emptiness triggers craving, and the addicted person attempts to make him- or herself whole through consumption. The experience of craving, a kind of psychological suffering, is a hallmark of addictions. In fact, it is such an integral part that the *Diagnostic and Statistical Manual of Mental Health Disorders* (5th ed.) explicitly acknowledges the possibility of lifelong craving and excludes this symptom from remission criteria.

Mindfulness deficits in individuals suffering from substance-use disorders have been consistently documented in the research literature.[13] The "thinking mind," always wanting, judging, comparing, and reacting to life, leads to the pursuit of pleasure and attempts to avoid pain—both of which come through harmful attachments to substances on a kind of "hedonic treadmill."[14] If addiction is interpreted as lack of presence, then mindfulness is the antidote. Through learning how to change the way they react to discomfort (be it physical, psychological, or emotional), people become able to create the space necessary to explore sensations with curiosity and acceptance rather than thoughtlessly attempting to snuff them out by using a substance.

Mindfulness-Based Relapse Prevention

One of the most well-known and empirically tested applications of mindfulness to addiction is Bowen, Chawla, and Marlatt's mindfulness-based relapse prevention (MBRP).[15] MBRP combines mindfulness meditation with traditional, cognitive-behavioral relapse prevention. It was initially inspired by Buddhist psychology and *vipassana* meditation. The program consists of a standardized eight-week curriculum that works as an adjunctive therapy and is intended for people who have completed treatment and are reasonably motivated for recovery. These authors describe this work as an attempt to balance self-discipline and compassion, a "middle way" between "harmful indulgence" and "strict renunciation." Drawing from Buddhism's "four noble truths," MBRP conceptualizes addiction as one manifestation of the suffering caused by attachment and craving. Like other mindfulness-based interventions, MBRP aims to help people respond to the urges and discomfort by instead learning to live with them.

The MBRP program manual outlines each of the weekly, two-hour-long sessions. Sessions build on one another, with topics unfolding as follows: automatic pilot and relapse, awareness of triggers and craving, mindfulness in daily life, mindfulness in high-risk situations, acceptance and skillful action, seeing thoughts as thoughts, self-care and lifestyle balance, and social support and continuing practice. The structured protocol for each session begins with an experiential mindfulness exercise followed by teaching and discussion. Exercises include the body scan, visualization of triggers, and mindful walking, among others. The treatment manual includes handouts and worksheets, and members are expected to engage in home practice between sessions. Studies have demonstrated MBRP's ability to reduce cravings and substance use.[16] While there are many areas of agreement between MBRP and traditional 12-step recovery (e.g., acceptance, letting go, importance of prayer/meditation), there are several points of divergence. These include endorsement of the disease model of addiction, labeling people as "addicts" or "alcoholics," and prioritizing abstinence as the ultimate goal.

Twelve-Step Facilitation

Twelve-Step Facilitation is a manualized, empirically supported treatment for substance-use disorders.[17] It was one of three treatments included in the federally funded, eight-year Project MATCH study that compared treatments for alcohol-use disorders. Despite its reliance on 12-step programs, TSF is not intended to replace free peer-support recovery with professional help. Rather, the primary goal of this treatment is to encourage active client participation in 12-step programs.

The 12-Step Model

All the various 12-step programs take their basic structure from the original one, Alcoholics Anonymous (AA). AA originated in the 1930s under the guidance of Bill Wilson and Dr. Bob Smith, who themselves struggled with drinking problems. The core assumption underlying the 12-step model is that addiction is both a medical and spiritual disease for which there is no cure. If left untreated, this progressive illness will only become worse. Moreover, self-knowledge and insight alone are not enough to produce change; the individual must have a "spiritual awakening" if he is to achieve lasting recovery. Much of AA's conceptualization of addiction came from earlier religious temperance organizations like the Oxford Group.[18] Originally a member of this group himself, Bill Wilson experienced a "white light" vision while hospitalized and wrote that he experienced the presence of God. He never drank again. Following this, Wilson set about articulating this spiritual program of recovery and spreading the message to others through the AA program.

AA's basic program is laid out in the book *Alcoholics Anonymous: The Story of How Many Thousands of Men and Women Have Recovered from Alcoholism*, often referred to simply as the "Big Book."[19] At the core of this and all other 12-step programs are the steps themselves. The ultimate goal of "working the steps" is to achieve a "spiritual awakening." As such, each step has a specific purpose in this overall process. Steps one to three are commonly referred to as the "surrender steps," marking the transition between the "self-will" of active addiction to acceptance, hope, and humility. Step four involves the creation of a detailed moral inventory that identifies "defects of character." Step five is sharing (i.e., confessing) this inventory with God and another person. Steps six and seven involve becoming willing and asking God to remove these "character defects." Steps eight and nine entail listing people and institutions that were harmed in the course of addiction and then making amends for these harms. Finally, steps 10 to 12 involve continuing to take personal inventory and expanding one's sense of spirituality through prayer and meditation. They also include being of service to others. These final steps are considered the "maintenance steps" because they are supposed to be practiced on a daily basis for the remainder of one's life.

Kelly and colleagues[20] found that AA participation was associated with increased spiritual practices, which partially mediated the relationship between meeting attendance and decreased alcohol use. Those who began treatment with lower levels of spirituality had larger increases in spiritual practices. Furthermore, spirituality was found to be a stronger factor for those with more severe alcohol problems, suggesting that the program works differently depending on the individual.

The 12-Step Facilitation Program

Twelve-Step Facilitation regards active engagement in the 12-step program as the main factor responsible for recovery. TSF formalizes the process by which people engage in recovery according to the 12-step program; it does not professionalize peer support. This treatment is divided into three components: The core program is used with all clients and consists of four topics—assessment of the client's substance-use problem and motivation for change, acceptance of powerlessness and unmanageability, surrender to a higher power, and getting active in AA or NA. The elective program is used with clients who are established in recovery and who have high levels of motivation. Topics include enabling, emotions, relationships, and the creation of a genogram. Finally, the conjoint program is for clients and significant others; it addresses enabling and detaching. Nowinsky and Baker[17] note that TSF has two primary goals: acceptance and surrender. The spiritual objectives of TSF are to increase hope that addiction can be arrested, develop belief and trust in a higher power, acknowledge character defects and past harms, and decrease shame and guilt associated with these by sharing with another person. These objectives follow steps one to five, and it is common for individuals to complete these steps while in treatment.

TSF is delivered in hour-long individual sessions over 12 to 15 weeks for the core program. Additional activities include journaling, keeping a log of meetings attended, and reading AA/NA literature. In keeping with 12-step program practices, counselors present these as "suggestions," not required assignments. Clients are also encouraged to utilize their sponsors and peer supports rather than professionals.

Prayer

Prayer is a common spiritual practice used by members of many different religions as well as those who do not identify with a specific faith. Sperry describes it as "the most distinctive and characteristically spiritual of all activities associated with the spiritual dimension" (p. 203).[10] In basic terms, prayer is a form of spiritual expression in which an individual or group seeks to communicate with the Divine. When used in the context of psychotherapy, prayer can increase client hope and comfort, enhance the therapeutic alliance, and combat isolation or loneliness. In addiction-specific treatment, prayer can increase readiness for change by stimulating self-reflection and help the individual articulate his or her motivations for recovery. This may involve shifting from what the individual wants to what he or she believes God wants for him or her.

Types of Prayer Used in Addiction Treatment

There are a number of different types of prayer associated with addiction treatment and recovery. These include mindfulness prayer, ritual prayer, and intercessory prayer. Centering prayer is a form of mindfulness prayer based on the ancient Christian practices of the desert fathers and mothers.[10,21]

Centering prayer involves choosing a sacred word or symbol to represent God's presence. The individual sits quietly (typically for 20 minutes, twice per day) and uses the symbol or word to maintain focus. Unlike Buddhist mindfulness interventions, the purpose of centering prayer is to awaken one's relationship with God rather than simply observe the present moment. Centering prayer also places less emphasis on physical considerations like posture or breathing. For those in recovery from substance-use disorders, this form of prayer can lead to the benefits of other mindfulness interventions while also enhancing one's relationship with a higher power.

Many spiritual and religious services include some form of ritual prayer. In addiction treatment and the broader recovery community, ritual prayers are common before and after meetings and groups. The Serenity Prayer and Lord's Prayer are common examples. In the context of recovery groups, ritual prayer can bring members together toward a shared purpose. Intercessory prayer is intended to produce healing and has been used in the treatment of physical and psychological ailments since the 19th century.[10] In treatment, this may involve the clinician praying directly with the client, allowing the client to pray while remaining silent, or praying for the client outside of treatment. For many people in recovery, praying for others and requesting prayers in return is a common practice.

Research on Prayer in Addiction Treatment

It is difficult to research the effectiveness of prayer because it is often one component of other treatment interventions, as in the case of Twelve-Step Facilitation. Some studies have attempted to examine prayer as an independent intervention. Walker and colleagues[22] conducted a randomized control pilot study investigating the effects of intercessory prayer on clients in inpatient treatment. They found that having other people pray for the client did not decrease alcohol consumption; however, prayer by the patients themselves was associated with decreased drinking frequency. Washington and Moxley[23] investigated the use of prayer in group therapy. They found that participants' prayers addressed a wide range of concerns, such as dealing with adversity and family responsibility, and that prayer led to increased clarity, hope, and motivation. Finally, in a series of four different randomized control studies, Lambert and colleagues[24] explored the relationship between prayer and alcohol consumption. They found that the frequency of prayer was negatively associated with alcohol use and alcohol-related problems even when controlling for participant variables. Participants in the prayer groups drank about half the amount of alcohol as the control groups. The researchers speculate that prayer might work by helping users "escape from the burden of the self" (p. 217),[24] which they previously accomplished through substance use.

Spiritual Assessment in Addiction Treatment

Clinicians who wish to provide spiritually oriented psychotherapy to clients with addictions should also be knowledgeable about spiritual assessment. According to Sperry,[10] an in-depth spiritual assessment is indicated under four circumstances: (1) when the client indicates that religious or spiritual issues are important, (2) when a spiritual issue is evident in the presenting problem(s), (3) when the clinical picture involves morality or guilt, and (4) when a concern about purpose in life is present. While many clients presenting with addiction may certainly fall within the first two categories, arguably all of them grapple with issues surrounding guilt and purpose.

Spiritual assessment can be conducted via structured/semistructured interviews and through the use of psychometric instruments. Important areas to address include the client's spiritual history, God image, spiritual beliefs and practices, spiritual identity, and level of involvement in a spiritual and/or religious community. Questions such as "How do you see God?" and "What role does your substance use play in your religious/spiritual practice?" help clarify the client's needs and challenges in these areas. Because of the widespread discussion of spiritual issues in addiction treatment and the recovery community, it is important that clinicians use spiritual assessment even when spirituality may not be the main focus of treatment.

Lawrence's God Image Inventory (GII)[25] was designed to measure God representations, or the way in which a person views God. This inventory and the theory underlying it assumes that individuals project certain characteristics onto their image of God. God representations can range from loving and caring to stern, vengeful, or indifferent. Transformative experiences such as initiating recovery from addiction and successful psychotherapy have been shown to improve a person's God image. This 156-item instrument has eight subscales that measure various aspects of one's perceived relationship with God. For example, the acceptance subscale refers to the degree to which a person feels worthy of God's love. Clinicians can administer the GII multiple times over the course of treatment to assess change.

The Higher Power Relationship Scale (HPRS)[26] measures the degree to which a person feels connected to his or her higher power and is based on 12-step philosophy. The 17-item HPRS is scored on a five-point Likert-type scale according to degree of belief. All items begin with the prompt "My Higher Power," and items include statements like "protects me," "guides me," and "is my friend." The Spiritual Belief Scale (SBS)[27] is an eight-item instrument based on the spiritual concepts found in Alcoholics Anonymous literature: gratitude, tolerance, humility, and release. Items include "I feel it is important to thank God when I manage to do the right thing" (gratitude) and "I know that forgiving those who have hurt me is important for my spiritual health" (tolerance).

Crumbaugh and Maholick's Purpose in Life test (PIL)[28] is a 20-item scale used to measure the extent to which people find their lives meaningful and purposeful. Lack of meaning and purpose has been consistently associated with substance abuse. PIL items assess a wide range of issues, including levels of boredom and despair, pleasure in daily tasks, and suicidal ideation. The Five Facet Mindfulness Questionnaire[29] is a 39-item instrument that measures five factors associated with mindfulness: observing, describing, acting with awareness, nonjudging of inner experience, and nonreactivity to inner experience. All these instruments can be used on intake to establish baselines and identify potential problem areas. They can also be used as outcome measures throughout the course of treatment.

Clinical Considerations

Clinicians would do well to anticipate how clients presenting with addictions are likely to respond to spiritual interventions. Here, there are two main considerations: first, the therapeutic relationship and transference/countertransference, and second, spirituality-related client resistance, which comes in many forms.

The alliance between clinician and client is a significant factor in treatment outcomes. In the context of spiritually oriented psychotherapy, this relationship requires new considerations. As noted in Sperry, "the therapeutic relationship can and does reflect a client's previous spiritual experiences" (p. 140).[10] Clients may transfer a range of thoughts, feelings, and expectations onto the clinician, as an authority figure, in much the same way they do with their images of God. Exploring the client's relationship (or lack thereof) with a higher power can yield valuable information about how the client is likely to respond to the clinician. For example, the client may have been raised in a conservative religious tradition that emphasized morality and depicts God as a harsh judge. This client is likely to feel ashamed and criticized about his or her substance use. When the clinician discusses spirituality, it may trigger these feelings, prompting the client to respond with anger, passivity, or other emotions. In contrast, clinicians' own spiritual/religious beliefs and values may influence how they perceive and treat clients. Substance use and related behaviors (e.g., illegal activities, lying) carry strong moral injunctions against them. Clinicians must be mindful of their own beliefs and reactions to client behavior so they do not undermine the therapeutic relationship. Clients who feel criticized, whether real or imagined, are not likely to be willing to explore sensitive issues.

Client resistance to discussing spirituality and participating in spiritual interventions is another consideration. This can happen for different reasons. Sometimes it is simply too early in treatment; the client may be in crisis, may have more immediate concerns like housing or legal problems, or may not yet trust the clinician. In this case, the clinician can collect relevant information as part of the overall assessment and case-conceptualization process and wait for a more appropriate time. Another possible reason for client resistance is confusion or skepticism about the role of spirituality in treatment. The client may question the need to discuss family religious background, thoughts about God, or other related topics, unsure of how they relate to presenting problems. In this case, clinicians should show empathy for the client's hesitation by taking it slow and educating the client about research evidence supporting this approach. Clients who have participated in addiction treatment or mutual-aid groups previously will typically be familiar with spirituality as a component of treatment. If a client is outwardly hostile toward spirituality and/or religion, the clinician should attempt to identify the reasons behind this reaction while still remaining respectful of the client's feelings. Ultimately, it is the client's choice whether or not to participate, though the clinician can explain and encourage.

A final form of resistance is when clients use spirituality as a means of avoiding problems or making changes. This is commonly called "spiritual bypass."[30] Clients may appear deeply committed to spiritual exploration and enthusiastically engage in spiritual interventions; upon investigation, however, this commitment is found to be superficial and designed to protect the client from the emotional discomfort of change. For example, a client with a dependent personality style may avoid interpersonal conflict by repeating the well-known recovery slogan "Let go, let God" instead of facing the conflict directly. Others applaud this client for being "spiritual," when in fact this behavior is designed to protect the client's maladaptive pattern. Clients engaged in spiritual bypass are not likely to be consciously aware of it, so the clinician's task is to raise their awareness without assuming that they are being intentionally deceitful or evasive.

Case Vignette

Jason is a 28-year-old Caucasian male who entered outpatient treatment through a court diversion program following a DUI arrest. He was suspicious and combative during the initial evaluation, stating that he does not "need anyone's help" and blaming the "heartless judge" for his current problems. Jason reported an extensive history of problem alcohol use beginning in late adolescence, including two previous arrests for public intoxication and numerous physical fights while drunk. He recently lost his retail job for arguing with his supervisor. Jason is single and lives alone. He has one male friend with whom he maintains a superficial relationship revolving around watching sports and drinking. Jason is an only child from a middle-class family. He revealed that his father also had problems with alcohol and died in a drinking-and-driving accident when Jason was eight years old. His mother died from cancer a few years later, when Jason was 12. Following this, Jason reports that his grandmother sent him to live in a boarding school until age 18.

Jason was guarded in response to the clinician's questions about his religious background and only provided information after he was assured that it was a standard part of the assessment process. He reported that he was raised Roman Catholic and attended church weekly with his family until moving away. Jason described a capricious image of God, seeing himself as the object of arbitrary torment. He repeatedly stated, "God hates me," citing the loss of his parents and current legal problems as evidence. Noting Jason's recent job loss and lack of social support, the clinician administered the Purpose in Life test. The results suggested that Jason feels alienated by others and frustrated by his inability to achieve his goals. He expressed a lifelong dream to attend college for creative writing but admitted that his drinking has made this impossible. Jason reported that he drinks when he feels overwhelmed and angry. He revealed that his DUI arrest occurred shortly after the conflict with his supervisor for which he was fired. "I just see red and reach for the bottle."

Following the assessment, the clinician concluded that spiritual interventions were indicated. Jason has experienced significant loss and consciously directs much of his anger toward God. Furthermore, his lack of engagement with life (i.e., friends, school) has led to feelings of hopelessness, and he uses alcohol to self-medicate. Jason's automatic response to negative emotions—drinking—suggests that he is unable to manage cravings. The clinician collaborates with Jason to develop a treatment plan that includes both secular and spiritual interventions. In addition to cognitive-behavioral interventions, Jason agrees to attend AA meetings and process his experiences there in therapy sessions. To help build distress tolerance, the clinician also teaches Jason mindfulness skills, including walking meditation and urge surfing. The clinician also suggested prayer as a way for Jason to reflect on his recovery and relationship with God; however, Jason stated that he was too angry and would not "give in like that."

As time goes on, Jason develops new friendships at AA meetings and widens his social support network. He attends recreational events and regularly eats dinner with members of his home group. While he experiences occasional relapses, these are brief, and he is able to identify the specific triggers behind them. In many cases, he identifies when he is feeling angry in the moment and does not drink. Initially, Jason tests the clinician by being rude or accusing the clinician of not caring. Eventually, however, the therapeutic alliance shifts and Jason expresses gratitude for this trusting, stable relationship. Jason's image of God undergoes a similar transformation. While in the beginning he often accuses God of "hating" him in response to stressful situations, he later describes God in more benevolent terms, using the language of "higher power" he learns in AA. Jason begins praying in the morning and at night at the suggestion of his sponsor. In therapy, Jason processes the deaths of his parents and his feelings of anger related to this perceived abandonment. Together with the clinician, he creates a new personal narrative of resilience and overcoming adversity rather than divine punishment. Toward the end of treatment, Jason takes the risk of applying to college.

References

1. McCabe, I. (2015). *Carl Jung and Alcoholics Anonymous: The twelve steps as a spiritual journey of individuation.* London, UK: Karnac Books.

2. Substance Abuse and Mental Health Services Administration. (2015). *National Survey of Substance Abuse Treatment Services (N-SSATS): 2014. Data on substance abuse treatment facilities.* BHSIS Series S-79, HHS Publication No. (SMA) 16-4963. Rockville, MD: Substance Abuse and Mental Health Services Administration.

3. Substance Abuse and Mental Services Administration. (2016). *Eight dimensions of wellness.* Retrieved on March 12, 2018, from https://www.samhsa.gov /wellness-initiative/eight-dimensions-wellness

4. Center for Substance Abuse Treatment. (2016). *Addiction counseling competencies: The knowledge, skills, and attitudes of professional practice.* Technical Assistance Publication (TAP). Series 21. HHS Publication No. (SMA) 15-4171. Rockville, MD: Substance Abuse and Mental Health Services Administration.

5. James, W. (1983). *The varieties of religious experience.* London, England: Penguin Classics.

6. Miller, W. R. (2016). Sacred cows and greener pastures: Reflections from 40 years in addiction research. *Alcoholism Treatment Quarterly, 34*(1), 92–115. doi:10.1080/07347324.2015.1077637

7. Miller, W. R. (2003). Spirituality, treatment and recovery. In M. Galanter (Ed.), *Recent developments in alcoholism: Vol. 16. Research on alcoholism treatment* (pp. 391–404). New York: Plenum Press.

8. Miller, W. M. (1998). Researching the spiritual dimensions of alcohol and other drug problems. *Addiction, 93*(7), 979–990.

9. Sussman, S., Milam, J., Arpawong, T. E., Tsai, J., Black, D. S., & Wills, T. A. (2013). Spirituality in addictions treatment: Wisdom to know . . . what it is. *Substance Use and Misuse, 48,* 1203–1217. doi:10.3109/10826084.2013.800343

10. Sperry, L. (2012). *Spirituality in clinical practice: Theory and practice of spiritually oriented psychotherapy* (2nd ed.). New York: Routledge.

11. Kabat-Zinn, J. (1994). *Wherever you go, there you are: Mindfulness meditation in everyday life.* New York: Hyperion.

12. Sperry, L., & Stoupas, G. (2017). Incorporating mindfulness in secular and spiritually oriented psychotherapy: Ethical concerns. *Spirituality in Clinical Practice, 4*(2), 152–154. doi:10.1037/scp0000132

13. Shorey, R. C., Brasfield, H., Anderson, S., & Stuart, G. L. (2014). Mindfulness deficits in a sample of substance abuse treatment seeking adults: A

descriptive investigation. *Journal of Substance Use, 19*(1), 194–198. doi:10.3109/14659891.2013.770570

14. Peltz, L., & Black, D. S. (2014). The thinking mind as addiction: Mindfulness as antidote. *Substance Use and Misuse, 49,* 605–607. doi:10.3109/10826084.2014.852803

15. Bowen, S., Chawla, N., & Marlatt, G. A. (2011). *Mindfulness-based relapse prevention for addictive disorders: A clinician's guide.* New York: Guilford Press.

16. Bowen, S., Chawla, N., Collins, S. E., Witkiewitz, K., Hsu, S., Grow, J., . . . Marlatt, G. A. (2009). Mindfulness-based relapse prevention for substance use disorders: A pilot efficacy trial. *Substance Abuse, 30*(4), 295–305. doi:10.1080/08897070903250084

17. Nowinsky, J., & Baker, S. (2003). *The twelve-step facilitation handbook: A systemic approach to recovery from substance dependence.* Center City, MN: Hazelden.

18. White, W., & Laudet, A. (2006). Spirituality, science and addiction counseling. *Counselor Magazine, 7*(1), 56–59.

19. Alcoholics Anonymous. (2001). *Alcoholics anonymous: The story of how many thousands of men and women have recovered from alcoholism* (4th ed.). New York: A. A. World Services.

20. Kelly, J. F., Stout, R. L., Magill, M., Tonigan, J. S., & Pagano, M. E. (2011). Spirituality in recovery: A lagged mediational analysis of Alcoholics Anonymous' principal theoretical mechanism of behavior change. *Alcoholism: Clinical and Experimental Research, 35*(3), 454–463. doi:10.1111/j.1530-0277.2010.01362.x

21. Blanton, P. G. (2011). The other mindful practice: Centering prayer and psychotherapy. *Pastoral Psychology, 60,* 133–147. doi:10.1007/s11089-010-0292-9

22. Walker, S. R., Tonigan, J. S., Miller, W. M., Corner, S., & Kahlich, L. (1997). Intercessory prayer in the treatment of alcohol abuse and dependence: A pilot investigation. *Alternative Therapies in Health and Medicine, 3*(6), 79–86.

23. Washington, O. G. M., & Moxley, D. P. (2001). The use of prayer in group work with African American women recovering from chemical dependency. *Families in Society, 82*(1), 49–59.

24. Lambert, N. M., Fincham, F. D., Stillman, T. F., & Marks, L. D. (2010). Invocations and intoxication: Does prayer decrease alcohol consumption? *Psychology of Addictive Behaviors, 24*(2), 209–219. doi:10.1037/a0018746

25. Lawrence, R. T. (1997). Measuring the image of God: The god image inventory and the god image scales. *Journal of Psychology and Theology, 25*(2), 214–226.

26. Rowan, N. L., Faul, A. C., Cloud, R. N., & Huber, R. (2006). The higher power relationship scale: A validation. *Social Work Practice and the Addictions, 6,* 81–96. doi:10.1300/J160v06n03_07

27. Schaler, J. A. (1996). Spiritual thinking in addiction treatment providers: The spiritual belief scale. *Alcoholism Treatment Quarterly, 14,* 7–33.

28. Crumbaugh, J., & Maholick, L. (1964). An experimental study of existentialism: The psychometric approach to Frankl's concept of noogenic neurosis. *Journal of Clinical Psychology, 20,* 200–207.

29. Baer, R. A., Smith, G. T., Hopkins, J., Krietemeyer, J., & Toney, L. (2006). Using self-report assessment methods to explore facets of mindfulness. *Assessment, 13*, 27–45. doi:10.1177/1073191105283504

30. Cashwell, C. S., Bentley, P. B., & Yarborough, J. P. (2007). The only way out is through: The peril of spiritual bypass. *Counseling and Values, 51*, 139–148.

CHAPTER SEVENTEEN

Using a Spiritually Sensitive Approach to Treat Problematic Pornography Consumption

Anthony Isacco, Domenick Tirabassi, Kelsey Porada, and Kate A. Meade

Caleb is a 27-year-old college-educated male, who decided to attend psychotherapy to decrease his long-standing anxiety. Caleb attributed most of his distress to the pressures of his work demands and relationship challenges with his spouse of three years, Jessica. Caleb and Jessica are both practicing Christians who attend services weekly and participate in a community Bible study offered through their church. As psychotherapy progresses, Caleb reveals that he watches pornography but that he would like to stop.

Have you ever encountered someone like Caleb? The Internet has contributed to a rise in pornography consumption due to factors such as anonymous browsing, affordability, and accessibility.[1] Pornography consumption has been correlated with a number of negative outcomes, including impairments in interpersonal, financial, and occupational functioning; emotional distress; and sexual dissatisfaction.[2] Studies in the United States and European countries (e.g., Denmark and Sweden) have found that males are exposed to pornography at younger ages and consume more pornography compared to females.[3] These negative outcomes, combined with the increased consumption of pornography particularly among males, suggest that mental health practitioners (shortened to *practitioners* for the remainder of this chapter) will likely encounter more pornography-related issues in psychotherapy.

Related to the case of Caleb, researchers have found that individuals with higher religiosity are more likely to experience emotional distress in relation to their pornography consumption.[4] If you are working with Caleb, what other information would you want to know about him before proceeding? What interventions are important to consider to help someone like Caleb? This chapter will continue to discuss Caleb—a composite, fictionalized client based on many similar clients that we have worked with over the years. This chapter describes a spiritually sensitive approach to assessment and psychotherapy that can be used to treat problematic pornography consumption (PPC) with religiously inclined clients like Caleb.

What Is Problematic Pornography Consumption?

The psychological literature about pornography consumption is often confusing to read given the many debates, various definitions, and mixed findings. We do not have space to review all those issues, but we briefly review some common points of confusion and offer our definition of PPC that we will use in subsequent sections of the chapter. The debate over whether pornography is morally "good" or "bad" has complicated the conceptual clarity of the construct. Psychologists and psychiatrists have been reluctant to overpathologize sexual behavior that may be considered "within normal limits." For some religiously inclined clients, such as Caleb, PPC has strong moral implications because viewing pornography is counter to his religious beliefs and practices. The perceived morality of the sexual behavior may exacerbate the experienced distress while also serving as a motivator to make positive changes. Concerns about PPC have been increasingly expressed by nonreligious/secular individuals and groups as well as federal and state governments over the past 5 to 10 years due to the evident negative outcomes associated with PPC. Rather than labeling pornography consumption as a moral issue, PPC has been labeled a public health crisis.

Practitioners will not find PPC as a specific diagnosis in the *Diagnostic and Statistical Manual of Mental Disorders* (5th ed., DSM-5).[5] Numerous researchers suspected that pornography addiction would be a DSM-5 diagnosis, but there was a lack of consensus given mixed findings and poor conceptual clarity.[6] Indeed, most psychological research studies introduce the topic with a neutral statement about the "positive and negative outcomes" associated with pornography consumption.[7] A psychiatric diagnosis is typically associated with negative outcomes; for example, we have yet to read a study linking major depressive disorder with positive outcomes. Given the mixed findings, some psychological researchers consider the impact of pornography

Table 17.1   Terms and Definitions

Term	Definition
Problematic Pornography Consumption[4]	Can be triggered, is persistent and intrusive, and influenced by powerful urges/impulses that are difficult to stop or control. PPC likely impacts at least one of the following domains: legal/occupational, social, physical, other pain, financial, and psychological/spiritual.[4]
Problematic Use of Internet Pornography[23]	Frequent to the point of excess or compulsion, triggered by an urge and difficult to control, aimed at attaining a positive emotional state or escaping a negative emotional state, and continues despite adverse consequences and personal distress and/or impairment.[23]
Pornography Addiction[24]	Pornography consumption that is addictive in the neurological sense: impacting the motivation, reward, and memory systems of the brain.[24]
Internet Sex Addiction[1]	Recurrent, intrusive sexual fantasies or urges, and the compulsion to repeatedly engage in sexual behaviors to cope, despite a detrimental impact on the individual's life.[1]
Hypersexual Disorder[6]	Any sexual behavior that one feels cannot be controlled and negatively impacts their life.[6]
Nonparaphilic Hypersexual Behavior[25]	Nonparaphilic sexual fantasies that are intense, recurring, and lead to negative consequences and significant distress, that impair an individual in one or more areas of functioning.[25]
Perceived Pornography Addiction[7]	The feeling that pornography usage is compulsive or out of control, and an inability to stop, despite the experience of severe or significant consequences.[7]
Compulsive Use of Internet-Based Sexually Explicit Material[26]	Characterized by difficulty keeping oneself from accessing sexually explicit material (SEM) online, despite the intention to stop, thinking about and looking forward to the material when not engaged with it, neglecting to complete important life tasks or obligations because of SEM, or preferring SEM to spending time with significant others.[26]
Compulsive Sexual Behavior[27]	Persistent and repetitive sexual impulses or urges that become a central focus of an individual's life, which they feel they cannot resist or control, and leads to feelings of distress and the neglecting of self-care and personal responsibility.[27]

(continued)

Table 17.1 *(continued)*

Sexual Dysfunction Unspecified[5]	302.70 (F52.9)
	Issues of sexual functioning that cause significant distress, but do not fit any other DSM-5 diagnoses relating to sexual function.[5]
Impulsive-Compulsive Internet Sexual Behavior[28]	Frequent and intrusive thoughts about sex and sexual behaviors, which an individual feels are out of control. This behavior is cyclic, triggered by an impulsive drive, and continued compulsively.[28]

consumption as a *perception* of the individual rather than an actual compulsion, addiction, and/or maladaptive behavior experienced by individuals.[7] Although not a formal diagnosis, practitioners have recognized the significant negative impact that PPC has had on their clients' lives and have diagnosed those clients with "sexual disorder, not otherwise specified." If not diagnosed, other researchers have suggested that PPC may be defined as a "clinical syndrome"—a bridge term that indicates a problem but not a diagnosis.[8] Table 17.1 includes a list of related terms and definitions. We aligned the chapter with the definition of PPC from Twohig, Crosby, and Cox,[4] which describes PPC as influenced by powerful urges/impulses that are difficult to stop or control and lead to some degree of functional impairment in at least one of the following domains: legal, occupational, social/interpersonal, physical, emotional, spiritual, and psychological. The definition is clinically useful across clients and settings because it avoids debate about the nature of the consumption and guides practitioners to address the functional difficulties with PPC in various life domains.

A Spiritually Sensitive Treatment Approach

To date, research on the treatment of PPC has been limited, and there are not any known evidence-based practices.[4] There has been some preliminary evidence for the use of motivational interviewing, cognitive-behavior therapy, and acceptance and commitment therapy for sexual compulsivity and pornography addiction. However, those therapies did not have religious/spiritual components to addressing PPC. There is not a religiously/spiritually based psychotherapy that has gone through experimentally controlled studies to determine its impact on PPC. Research on the integration of religious/spiritual constructs and tools in psychotherapy has advanced and is relevant to clients such as Caleb. Given the state of the treatment research for PPC, this chapter focuses on utilizing a spiritually sensitive approach to treatment.[9] Using technical terminology from Chambless and colleagues,[10] the clinical interventions in this chapter have "modest" research support, meaning that one or two well-designed studies support the efficacy of the intervention. The good news is that practitioners have more guidance in addressing PPC now than they did 5 to 10 years ago. We provide an overview of a four-phase spiritually sensitive approach—spiritual assessment, identification of spiritual needs or concerns, addressing those needs, and provision of mental health care with an integration of spirituality.[9] This section describes how to implement the phases with PPC.

Phase 1: Assessment

As mentioned above, we are using the term PPC,[4] which is defined as powerful urges that are difficult to stop or control and lead to some functional impairment for the client. The PPC definition provides practitioners a starting point for assessment, which can inform the treatment process. The first part of the assessment is to gather information about the pornography consumption. Useful questions to ask during a clinical interview include the following:

1. **Frequency, quantity, and content:** How often do you view pornography? Assess the frequency of consumption (days per week and hours per day) as well as the pornographic content (e.g., pictures, videos, soft core, hard core).
2. **Control and inhibiting PPC efforts:** To what extent are you able to control or not control your pornography consumption? Do you want to stop viewing pornography? What have you tried to help you stop viewing pornography? What has been helpful and what has not been helpful? Assess impulse control, urges, and difficulty controlling the PPC.
3. **Functional impairment in a life domain:** What problems in your life are related to PPC? What problems in your life are triggering the PPC?

Caleb reported that he consumes pornography for approximately 90 minutes per day, five to seven days per week, which has been occurring for approximately one-and-a-half years. He expressed a sincere desire to stop viewing pornography and was frustrated with his inability to stop. Caleb described his unsuccessful attempts at stopping his PPC through intercessory prayer, "bouncing my eyes" to avoid alluring images of women, and exercise. Caleb was unable to identify any specific underlying motivations to his PPC because he wanted to stop and understood the behavior as contrary to his religious beliefs. Caleb has noticed feeling "terrible" about himself due to his PPC. In terms of possible contributing stressors, Caleb reported that the "honeymoon is over" in his marital relationship. He described increasing arguments with his wife over finances, household task distribution, and how to spend the holidays equally among their families. He identified increased work responsibilities and travel as a stressor in his profession as a pharmaceutical sales representative. He currently travels three or four days per week, compared to one or two days per week last year, and his sales quotas for his accounts have increased. The work travel and the shame associated with PPC have contributed to Caleb avoiding religious services on the weekends, which compounds his feelings of shame and sense of disconnection from God and his faith community.

The ability of individuals to talk openly about their sexual problems is important due to the often hidden and isolative nature of the problem. Stigma, shame, and guilt are just a few barriers to self-disclosures about PPC, particularly among religious/spiritual clients. Gender socialization may further inhibit male clients from overly verbose descriptions of PPC with a practitioner. Despite the importance of assessment using open-ended questions within the clinical interview, it is likely that discussing PPC is difficult for clients like Caleb. It can be helpful to administer brief, self-report scales to gather additional information that sheds light on the scope, level of distress, varying degrees of risk, specific behaviors, and motivations of PPC that might not readily be disclosed during the clinical interview. We recommend three scales.

The Internet Sex Screening Test[11] is a 34-item, self-report assessment of problematic sexual feelings, behaviors, and compulsions on the Internet. Scores can range from 0 to 25. Scores ranging from 1 to 8 indicate "low risk," 9 to 18 indicate "at-risk" sexual behavior, and 19 and above indicate high-risk sexual behavior and the likelihood of corresponding impairment in some areas of life. The Pornography Consumption Inventory (PCI) is a 15-item, self-report assessment of motivations for pornography consumption. The PCI assesses four motivations: (1) emotional avoidance, (2) sexual curiosity, (3) excitement seeking, and (4) sexual pleasure. Scores can range from 15 to 75, with higher scores indicating greater tendencies to use pornography, per the four motivations. The Hypersexual Behavior Inventory (HBI-19) is a 19-item, self-report assessment of sexual fantasies, urges, behaviors, thoughts, and feelings that may be problematic and cause distress. Scores can range from 19 to 95, with a score of 53 or above indicative of problematic hypersexual behavior.

Caleb scored a 10 on the ISST, indicating "at-risk" sexual behavior. Specific behaviors that he endorsed included "I repeatedly attempt to stop certain sexual behaviors and fail" and "I hide some of my sexual behaviors from others." Caleb scored a 50 on the PCI, with his score reflective of items that compose the emotional avoidance motivation factor (i.e., he uses pornography to avoid negative and uncomfortable emotions). Some items that he endorsed included "I turn to it [pornography] when I'm feeling down, sad, or lonely" and "I use it [pornography] to change my mood when I am anxious, stressed, or angry." Caleb scored a 56 on the HBI, which is above the cut-off of 53 and indicative of problematic hypersexual behavior. His HBI score endorsed problems with controlling his pornography use ("I do things sexually that are against my values and beliefs") and consequences ("My sexual activities interfere with aspects of my life such as work or school").

Phase 2: Identification of Spiritual Concerns

Taken together, Caleb's responses during the clinical interview and on the three self-report measures indicated problems associated with his pornography consumption, such as marital discord, maladaptive coping with negative emotions, and an inability to stop his sexual behavior on his own. Although he uses pornography to cope with negative emotions, the coping is temporary and results in increased anxiety. His spiritual concerns were identified as a negative God image, fear of punishment from God, moral browbeating, and interpersonal disconnection from his wife and religious community—all of which participate in a feedback loop and further exacerbate Caleb's struggles with coping, anxiety, and accessing social support.

Phase 3: Addressing PPC and the Associated Spiritual Concerns

Addressing PPC and the associated spiritual concerns is a two-part counseling process. First, we discuss how to address the spiritual concerns associated with PPC that we identified in the assessment phase (spiritual struggles, forgiveness). Second, we describe how practitioners can integrate empirically supported spiritual tools[12] in psychotherapy to address PPC and related psychological concerns (e.g., anxiety and interpersonal dysfunction).

Spiritual struggles arise when people experience difficulties that involve their faith beliefs. There are three main categories of spiritual struggle: divine, interpersonal, and intrapsychic.[13] Divine spiritual struggles encompass issues in one's relationship with the Divine. Intrapsychic spiritual struggles exemplify internal conflicts between one's thoughts, feelings, and faith beliefs. Interpersonal spiritual struggles occur when people have difficulties in relationships with other religious people in their lives. Clients who are experiencing spiritual struggles might report that they are questioning their faith, feeling disconnected from God, or disengaging in religious practices. One of the goals of spiritually sensitive treatment is to help clients identify and resolve spiritual struggles. Below is a sample of therapeutic dialogue between Caleb and his practitioner working to make the spiritual struggle explicit.

Practitioner: Earlier in the session, you mentioned that you were feeling disconnected from God. Can you tell me more about this disconnect?

Caleb: Yeah. Ever since I started watching porn, there is just this distance that I feel because I can't connect to God. I have been having a hard time praying and getting motivated to go to church.

Practitioner: So part of this disconnect is because you feel abandoned by God.

Caleb: I think that's what it comes down to. God is not there for me anymore. He abandoned me.

Once the spiritual struggle has been identified, the practitioner can spend some time exploring that specific issue with the client. Exploring the spiritual struggle helps to facilitate the client to resolve the spiritual struggle. It should be noted that resolving spiritual struggles is a process, and resolution occurs on a continuum, ranging from unresolved to fully resolved. There are three strategies for resolving a spiritual struggle: spiritual meaning making, transforming images of God, and resolving spiritual inconsistencies. Spiritual meaning making occurs when the client is able to make sense out of the spiritual struggle.[13] The practitioner assists by helping the client to take a wider and deeper perspective that refocuses the client on an adaptive meaning to the struggle. God images are affect-laden, mental representations of an individual's divine attachment figures (e.g., God, Buddha, Jesus, Shiva).[14] Transforming God images with a client experiencing a spiritual struggle entails helping the client reconnect with God by reframing the image of God from punishing, distant, or harsh, to loving, forgiving, and present. Spiritual inconsistencies are differences between a client's thoughts, feelings, and religious beliefs. To begin resolving these inconsistencies, a practitioner helps the client to understand the inconsistency and create a congruence between thoughts, feelings, and beliefs.

Below is a sample therapeutic dialogue with Caleb, illustrating how to resolve a spiritual struggle through spiritual meaning making.

Practitioner: You said these feelings that God had abandoned you started after you began watching pornography?

Caleb: Yeah. My faith was so strong, but then I was just overcome with feelings of loneliness. I never thought that I would feel abandoned by God.

Practitioner: I'm wondering if there is a deeper meaning to this struggle.

Caleb: I feel like this distance might be a wake-up call. I've been hiding from so many things and escaping into the fantasy world of pornography. Maybe God is letting me understand what it feels like to be truly alone and challenging me to be a more committed husband.

Phase 4: Integrating Spiritual Tools to Decrease PPC

Increased anxiety often triggers "experiential avoidance," or habitually distracting oneself from unpleasant feelings through PPC, which contributes to worsening problems.[15] Clients exhibiting experiential avoidance have not learned effective ways to cope with anxiety. Practitioners need to work with clients to substitute a positive coping skill to help dismantle a problematic coping mechanism. A variety of positive coping strategies exist; we focus on prayer as a spiritual tool that can be integrated into counseling. Equipping religious clients with the spiritual tool of prayer can prove beneficial in reducing anxiety, targeting a key trigger for PPC-related experiential avoidance.[16] Like other coping skills, the practice of prayer is a habit to develop and strengthen, even during times of relative calm. Some clients may have prayer preferences and could benefit from therapeutic encouragement and accountability. Other clients may not have a prayer regimen, and counseling can help them explore and identify a congruent prayer type. During Caleb's assessment, he indicated that he uses pornography to deal with anxiety. This dialogue illustrates how a practitioner can help Caleb identify prayer from his religious background to more effectively cope with anxiety associated with PPC.

> Practitioner: It may be worth considering how we can use your prayer to help you manage anxiety, so you can regain some peace and stay in control of your mind and body. This way, you won't have to rely on the porn videos.
>
> Caleb: Yeah. I really want that.
>
> Practitioner: Okay. We can start simple. Do you have any scripture verses you sometimes come back to that you've noticed help you feel better?
>
> Caleb: Well, actually, at one of our Wednesday-night services a while back, we reflected on this verse that went like, "The Lord is with me; I will not be afraid. What can man do to me? The Lord is with me. He is my helper." I repeated that to myself at work, but then I stopped.
>
> Practitioner: How would you feel when you'd repeat that verse to yourself?
>
> Caleb: Honestly, I would feel more in control. And afterward, even if it didn't go as well as I wanted it to, I'd still walk out thinking, "The Lord is with me," and it wouldn't be so bad.

Many individuals with PPC feel intense shame about their pornography use. Shame is worsened by rumination on painful ideas about oneself, such as one's sinfulness or failure. This shame crosses into the spiritual domain when it is linked to ideas of condemnation from God and necessitates forgiveness. The relationship between shame and PPC can be cyclic, in which shame begets use and more use begets more shame. Shame is a strong predictor of continued hypersexual behavior, which makes it a pertinent target for PPC treatment with Caleb.[17] Forgiveness is another efficacious component to a spiritually sensitive approach with Caleb to help reduce shame and increase self-compassion.[18] Examples include modifying his thought patterns that worsen shame and rumination, practicing mindful meditations on self-compassion, and helping Caleb reframe his understanding of God to a more positive image.

> Practitioner: I've heard you say you feel terrible about yourself, dirty, sinful. You have a lot of painful images and shame that you've been carrying with you for quite some time. But I'm wondering—where does forgiveness come into this?
>
> Caleb: I guess it really hasn't.
>
> Practitioner: It seems like you have shame that is really in need of forgiveness, both from God and from yourself. Living in shame hasn't been healthy for you.
>
> Caleb: No, it hasn't. I want to feel forgiven.

PPC often involves withdrawal from relationships. Social withdrawal, shame, and low self-esteem feed back into PPC.[19] Breaking the negative feedback loop between these interconnected issues is a primary therapeutic goal. For religious clients, fostering religious attendance might be an effective tool for decreasing PPC vis-à-vis increasing social connections.[12,20] However, a religious client's shame due to PPC may inhibit attendance at religious services. We see a similar pattern with Caleb. Caleb's avoidance of religious services is exacerbated by his irrational fears that people in his religious community will learn about his PPC. By reintegrating church attendance, the practitioner encourages the religious client's ability to engage in healthy relationships that alleviate distress and provide renewed support. Below is a sample of therapeutic dialogue between Caleb and the practitioner about increasing his attendance at religious services.

> Practitioner: You mentioned belonging to a church and enjoying going to services in the past. But now you don't. What's stopping you from going back?
>
> Caleb: I don't know. People might find out about my PPC. But, I guess it could be helpful. I used to get a lot out of going to services. It's something my wife and I did together.
>
> Practitioner: We've talked a lot recently about your feeling that you're struggling to connect with your wife. It sounds like maybe going back to church would be a way for you to get some support and feel closer to her. Can you commit to going this week with that intention?
>
> Caleb: I do think it would help Jessica and me. I can commit to doing that.

The practitioner encourages Caleb to consider the supportive aspects of his church attendance so he can participate in a shared activity that facilitates connection in his marriage. Throughout this process, it is important to consider how practitioners talk about church attendance and the moral struggles clients experience. The goal is not to invalidate the shame or guilt they feel but to encourage reengagement in sources of spiritual support that facilitate interpersonal connection and intimacy, which helps to decrease psychological correlates to PPC.

Cultural, Ethical, and Legal Issues

This chapter has illustrated that religious and spiritual issues intersect with PPC in ways that are salient to clinical practice. However, some practitioners are uncomfortable addressing PPC, avoid the topic, minimize the issue, and/or lack competence to help in this area. It is beyond the scope of this chapter to detail each religion's teachings related to pornography. We recognize that this is an overgeneralization, but it is rather safe to conclude that the major world religions (e.g., Christianity, Judaism, Islam, Mormonism, Catholicism) have teachings against pornography. Therefore, religious clients striving to live in accordance with their religion's teachings (such as Caleb) will be trying to stop their PPC. Therapy that attempts to reframe or abandon the client's faith beliefs and sexual morality will likely be ineffective and is not advised.[7]

Other practitioners may have strong feelings against pornography and overpathologize the problems. Both extremes often relate to the practitioner's own sense of morality and own religiosity of sexual behavior, which will likely interfere with positive therapeutic progress. Either way, practitioners need to avoid imposing their personal values on clients. Thus, we suggest that practitioners utilize the multicultural counseling competencies of self-awareness, cultural knowledge of the client's religious/spiritual worldview regarding PPC, and skills that are congruent with the client's religiosity/spirituality and targeted change. Such an approach represents an ethical integration of religious/spiritual issues relevant to the specific client's background, values, and worldview.

In terms of utilizing culturally congruent skills and interventions, this chapter illustrated the constellation of issues and concerns that PPC is situated within, which makes stopping the behavior that much more difficult. There is no silver-bullet treatment in the psychological literature. Thus, practitioners should be prepared to use many tools in the proverbial toolbox (Table 17.2). Please note that Table 17.2 is not an exhaustive list, we are not commercially endorsing any product, and the empirical support for these tools is variable. However, we have found that the resources can be helpful and easily integrated into PPC treatment with religious/spiritual clients.

Table 17.2 Additional Spiritual Resources and Tools for Religious Clients with PPC

Books

Every Man's Battle: This interactive workbook, from Stephen Arterburn, Fred Stoeker, and Mike Yorkey, is written from a Christian perspective and provides personal anecdotes and a detailed plan for refraining from pornography use. Part of a series.

Overcoming Pornography Addiction: A Spiritual Solution: This book, written by J. Brian Bransfield, provides information about pornography use in the context of Christianity, focusing on how to utilize spirituality to overcome pornography use.

Wired for Intimacy: This book, by William Struthers, describes the effects of pornography on the male brain. It articulates common assumptions surrounding pornography use and provides insights and discussion for both married and single Christian men.

Web sites

Integrity Restored: This Web site offers a seven-step model for overcoming pornography use, as well as support for spouses, parents, and clergy, within a Catholic framework. The site provides links to finding a therapist, events, seminars, and youth outreach programs. Integrity Restored also has a podcast and blog geared toward overcoming pornography.

The Porn Effect: This Web site focuses on helping individuals create a "Battle Plan" to overcome their pornography use. It provides a place to ask experts, from members of clergy to psychologists, as well as an online support, prayer, and story sharing board, and resources and events for middle school students to adults.

PornHelp: This Web site provides an unbiased overview of all possible ways to overcome pornography use, with a section on religious resources divided by religious denomination.

Purity Is Possible: This Web site, designed by psychiatrist Dr. Kevin Majeres, provides nine self-help modules focused on helping individuals align their sexual desires and actions with their ideals. A value-based curriculum that is not explicitly religious.

Reclaim Sexual Health: This Web site offers an anonymous, faith-based, low-cost recovery program with a Catholic focus that involves training, online journaling, daily tracking, coaching, and 24/7 support.

Accountability Software

Accountable2You: This accountability software works across devices to record, track, and monitor online activity while sending the information to accountability partners. It is designed to work with Web site filtering software. Requires a monthly fee.

(continued)

Table 17.2 *(continued)*

Covenant Eyes: This accountability and filtering software provides tracking of online activity, as well as filtering of selected content, and provides reports sent to accountability partners to help keep individuals on track. Requires a monthly fee.

X3 Watch: This accountability and filtering software offers a customizable choice of acceptable and unacceptable online content, as well as weekly and instant update e-mails sent to accountability partners based on content. Requires a yearly fee.

Apps

The Fighter App: This app utilizes objectives and badges to motivate users, as well as a "battle tracker" to keep track of successes and backslides. The app requires users to keep a regular journal and to document when, where, how, and their mood following a setback.

Overcome Porn 40 Day Challenge by Covenant Eyes: This 40-day app offers 40 separate lessons on using spirituality to overcome pornography use, as well as a place to track purity goals and progress.

Victory (LT): This app, created by Life Teen, is geared toward Catholic teens, and provides users with daily motivational quotes and connects them with accountability partners. Using a "temptation scale," the app aims to help users identify their triggers.

Other Spiritual, Non-Therapy Interventions

Spiritual Direction: This mentoring experience can be provided individually or in groups, and allows for a deep exploration of the spiritual self and how God plays a part in one's life.

Pastoral Counseling: This counseling service is offered by religious individuals with a knowledge of mental health issues, and integrates the fields of psychology and religion.

Confession: This Catholic sacrament of acknowledging one's sins to a priest is meant to help one obtain forgiveness for their sins.

Sex Addicts Anonymous: This twelve-step system focuses on men and women with a variety of sexual addictions, providing them with meetings and resources throughout the United States and other countries.

Sexual Recovery Anonymous: This twelve-step system focuses on individuals struggling with sexual compulsivity, with the goal of sexual sobriety. Meetings throughout the United States and a multitude of resources are available for free.

Child pornography is a primary legal issue with PPC. Whereas adult pornography is considered a legal form of personal expression in the United States, child pornography does not have the same designation and is illegal.[21] Child pornography is defined by producing, disseminating, viewing, and/or possessing pornographic material (e.g., images and videos) that includes children/minors under the age of 18 in a sexual act and may include sexual exploitation, abuse, and trafficking.[21] Many states (e.g., Pennsylvania) designate that creating, distributing, or *intentionally* viewing child pornography are offenses that mandate reporting.[22] Practitioners should be aware of mandated reporter laws for the state that they practice in, as child-pornography laws are rapidly changing. Practitioners practicing in states that mandate reporting for child pornography should include a statement on their informed consent document for clients about their role as a mandated reporter in response to disclosures about child pornography. PPC with adult pornography, although legal, can create functional impairment in the workplace through decreased productivity, distraction, fears of being caught, and loss of employment. Thus, practitioners can help clients understand their workplace policies about pornography consumption in the work setting and on work computers and the specific grounds for dismissal. Court cases in the United States (e.g., Wisconsin) and Canada (e.g., New Brunswick) have upheld the termination of an employee accessing pornography in the workplace.

Summary and Conclusions

PPC is associated with various negative outcomes across domains. Practitioners working with religious clients are guided to consider the moral, religious, and spiritual effects of PPC on their clients' functioning. In this chapter, we described a spiritually sensitive approach to treatment focused on four phases: assessment, identification, addressing the spiritual concerns, and spiritual integration with mental health counseling. Such an approach can be tailored to the unique cultural background and specific functional problems associated with PPC of each religious client. PPC is seemingly an ever-growing problem and considered a public health crisis. Practitioners are likely to encounter more clients with PPC and the associated spiritual, religious, psychological concerns.

References

1. Griffiths, M. D. (2012). Internet sex addiction: A review of empirical research. *Addiction Research and Theory, 20*(2), 111–124. doi:10.3109/16066359.2011.588351

2. Philaretou, A. G., Mahfouz, A. Y., & Allen, K. R. (2005). Use of Internet pornography and men's well-being. *International Journal of Men's Health, 4,* 149–169. doi:10.3149/jmh.0402.149

3. Regnerus, M. D., Gordon, D., & Price, J. (2016). Documenting pornography use in America: A comparative analysis of methodological approaches. *The Journal of Sex Research, 53,* 873–881. doi:10.1080/00224499.2015.1096886

4. Twohig, M. P., Crosby, J. M., & Cox, J. M. (2009). Viewing Internet pornography: For whom is it problematic, how, and why? *Sexual Addiction & Compulsivity, 16,* 253–266. doi:10.1080/10720160903300788

5. American Psychiatric Association. (2013). *Diagnostic and statistical manual of mental disorders: DSM-5.* Washington, DC: American Psychiatric Association.

6. Kafka, M. P. (2014). What happened to hypersexual disorder? *Archives of Sexual Behavior, 43,* 1259–1261. doi:10.1007/s10508-014-0326-y

7. Grubbs, J. B., Exline, J. J., Pargament, K. I., Volk, F., & Lindberg, M. J. (2017). Internet pornography use, perceived addiction, and religious/spiritual struggles. *Archives of Sexual Behavior, 46*(6), 1733–1745. doi:10.1007/s10508-016-0772-9

8. Karila, L., Wery, A., Weinstein, A., Cottencin, O., Petit, A., Reynaud, M., & Billieux, J. (2014). Sexual addiction or hypersexual disorder: Different terms for the same problem? A review of the literature. *Current Pharmaceutical Design, 20,* 1–9. doi:10.2174/13816128113199990619

9. Sperry, L. (2016). Varieties of religious and spiritual treatment: Spirituality oriented psychotherapy and beyond. *Spirituality in Clinical Practice, 3*(1), 1. doi:10.1037/scp0000097

10. Chambless, D. L., Baker, M. J., Baucom, D. H., Beutler, L. E., Calhoun, K. S., Crits-Christoph, P., . . . Woody, S. R. (1998). Update on empirically validated therapies: II. *The Clinical Psychologist, 51,* 3–16.

11. Delmonico, D. L., & Miller J. A. (2003). The Internet Sex Screening Test: A comparison of sexual compulsives versus non-sexual compulsives. *Sexual Relationship Therapy, 18,* 261–276. doi:10.1080/1468199031000153900

12. Plante, T. G. (2009). *Spiritual practices in psychotherapy: Thirteen tools for enhancing psychological health.* Washington, DC: American Psychological Association. doi:10.3109/01612840.2011.587939

13. Pargament, K. I. (2011). *Spiritually integrated psychotherapy: Understanding and addressing the sacred.* Chicago, IL: Guilford Press.

14. Davis, D. B., Moriarty, G. L., & Mauch, J. C. (2013). God images and god concepts: Definitions, development, and dynamics. *Psychology of Religion and Spirituality, 5*(1), 51–60.

15. Wetterneck, C. T., Burgess, A. J., Short, M. B., Smith, A. H., & Cervantes, M. E. (2012). The role of sexual compulsivity, impulsivity, and experiential avoidance in Internet pornography use. *Psychological Record, 62*(1), 3–17. doi:10.1007/BF03395783

16. Anderson, J. W., & Nunnelley, P. A. (2016). Private prayer associations with depression, anxiety and other health conditions: An analytical review of clinical studies. *Postgraduate Medicine, 128*(7), 635–641. doi:10.1080/00325481.2016.1209962

17. Reid, R. C. (2010). Differentiating emotions in a patient sample of hypersexual men. *Journal of Social Work Practice in the Addictions, 10*(2), 197–213. doi:10.1080/15332561003769369

18. Wade, N. G., Hoyt, W. T., Kidwell, J. E. M., & Worthington, E. L., Jr. (2014). Efficacy of psychotherapeutic interventions to promote forgiveness: A meta-analysis. *Journal of Consulting and Clinical Psychology, 82*(1), 154–170.

19. Wilt, J. A., Cooper, E. B., Grubbs, J. B., Exline, J. J., & Pargament, K. I. (2016). Associations of perceived addiction to Internet pornography with religious/spiritual and psychological functioning. *Sexual Addiction and Compulsivity, 23*(2–3), 260–278. doi:10.1080/10720162.2016.1140604

20. Hardy, S. A., Steelman, M. A., Coyne, S. M., & Ridge, R. D. (2013). Adolescent religiousness as a protective factor against pornography use. *Journal of Applied Developmental Psychology, 34*, 131–139. doi:10.1016/j.appdev.2012.12.002

21. Mapes, B. E. (2015). Child pornography and the law. *The Pennsylvania Psychologist Quarterly,* September.

22. Knapp, S., Baturin, R., & Tepper, A. M. (2015). Child pornography provisions under child protective services law. *Pennsylvania Psychology Quarterly,* September.

23. Kor, A., Zilcha-Mano, S., Fogel, Y. A., Mikulincer, M., Reid, R. C., & Potenza, M. N. (2014). Psychometric development of the problematic pornography use scale. *Addictive Behaviors, 39*, 861–868. doi:10.1016/j.addbeh.2014.01.027

24. Hilton, D. L., Jr. (2013). Pornography addiction – a supranormal stimulus considered in the context of neuroplasticity. *Socioaffective Neuroscience & Psychology, 3*, 1. doi:10.3402/snp.v3i0.20767

25. Hook, J. N., Reid, R. C., Penberthy, J. K., Davis, D. E., & Jennings, D. J. (2013). Methodological review of treatments for nonparaphilic hypersexual behavior. *Journal of Sex and Marital Therapy, 40*, 294–308. doi:10.1080/00926 23X.2012.751075

26. Downing, M. J., Antebi, N., & Schrimshaw, E. W. (2014). Compulsive use of Internet-based sexually explicit media: Adaptation and validation of the Compulsive Internet Use Scale (CIUS). *Addictive Behaviors, 39*, 1126–1130. doi:10.1016/j.addbeh.2014.03.007

27. Krueger, R. B. (2016). Diagnosis of hypersexual or compulsive sexual behavior can be made using ICD-10 and DSM-5 despite rejection of this diagnosis by the American Psychiatric Association. *Addiction, 111*(12), 2110–2111. doi:10.1111/add.13366

28. Mick, T. M., & Hollander, E. (2006). Impulsive-compulsive sexual behavior. *CNS Spectrums, 11*, 944–955. doi:10.1017/S1092852900015133

About the Editor and Contributors

Editor

Thomas G. Plante is the Augustin Cardinal Bea, S. J. University Professor and directs the Spirituality and Health Institute at Santa Clara University. He is also an adjunct clinical professor of psychiatry and behavioral sciences at Stanford University School of Medicine. He recently served as vice-chair of the National Review Board for the Protection of Children and Youth for the U.S. Conference of Catholic Bishops and is past president of the Society for the Psychology of Religion and Spirituality (Division 36) of the American Psychological Association. He has authored or edited 21 books, including most recently *Graduating with Honor: Best Practices to Promote Ethics Development in College Students* (Praeger, 2017), *The Psychology of Compassion and Cruelty: Understanding the Emotional, Spiritual, and Religious Influences* (Praeger, 2015), *Sexual Abuse in the Catholic Church: A Decade of Crisis, 2002–2012* (Praeger, 2011, with Kathleen L. McChesney), and *Spiritual Practices in Psychotherapy: Thirteen Tools for Enhancing Psychological Health* (2009). He has also published over 200 scholarly professional journal articles and book chapters. He teaches courses in abnormal psychology, health psychology, ethics in psychology, and the psychology of religion and spirituality and maintains a private clinical practice as a licensed psychologist in Menlo Park, California. He has published 10 edited or authored book projects with ABC-CLIO/Praeger since 1999.

Contributors

Jill E. Bormann is a clinical nurse specialist in adult psychiatric–mental-health nursing and a clinical professor at the Hahn School of Nursing and Health Sciences/Betty and Bob Beyster Institute for Nursing Research, Advanced Practice, and Simulation, University of San Diego. Over the past 18 years, Dr. Bormann and colleagues have led development and research on a complementary, mind-body-spirit intervention for symptom management and well-being—the Mantram Repetition Program—which has earned the EdgeRunner distinction for nursing innovation from the American Academy of Nursing.

Suzette Brémault-Phillips is an occupational therapist and associate professor in the Department of Occupational Therapy, Faculty of Rehabilitation Medicine, at the University of Alberta and holds a PhD in theology. Her research and teaching interests with military and civilian populations include medical rehabilitation; mental and spiritual health, well-being, fitness, and resilience; aging and complex needs; spiritual assessment; interprofessional collaboration; and competency enhancement. She is currently on a research team funded to study the health effects of the 2016 Alberta wildfires on pregnant women and their babies.

Barbara M. Burns is a professor of child studies at Santa Clara University and a developmental psychologist whose research is focused on promoting well-being and school readiness in young children from families facing adversity and economic disadvantage. Burns leads a family intervention program in San Jose, California, called Safe, Secure and Loved, which is based on the science of resilience and promotes attachment, executive function skills, and stress management in children and families.

Andrea L. Canada is a licensed psychologist and associate professor of psychology at Rosemead School of Psychology, Biola University. Her clinical and research interests focus on religious/spiritual well-being across the cancer survivorship continuum.

John T. Chirban is a clinical psychologist and is director of Cambridge Counseling Associates and lecturer in psychology within the Department of Psychiatry at Harvard Medical School. In 2003, he was named 40th Anniversary Senior Fellow at the Center for the Study of World Religions at Harvard University. In addition to several volumes, he authored *Collateral Damage: Guiding and Protecting Your Child through the Minefield of Divorce* (2017).

Don E. Davis is an associate professor of psychology at Georgia State University and has published over 160 articles and chapters and several books. He studies positive psychology with special emphasis on humility, forgiveness, and religious and spiritual issues.

Angela DiMartino is a program manager for Senior Vitality and Healthy Living Aftercare Group and several health-care improvement programs at Curry Senior Center in San Francisco. Ms. DiMartino conducts research on healthy aging programs for seniors and explores complementary and integrative modalities that incorporate exercise, nutrition, health coaching, and spirituality.

David B. Feldman is a professor of counseling psychology at Santa Clara University. His research concerns hope, meaning, and coping with highly negative events. He is the coauthor of *Supersurvivors: The Surprising Link between Suffering and Success* (2014) and two other books.

Lucy Finkelstein-Fox is a doctoral student in clinical psychology at the University of Connecticut. Ms. Finkelstein-Fox studies strategies for self-regulation and coping with stress as they affect mental and physical health.

Christina E. Fitch is an assistant professor of palliative medicine at UMass Medical School and works clinically at Baystate Medical Center. She teaches resiliency skills, expert communication in serious illness, and topics in global health.

Brandon J. Griffin is a research health science specialist at the San Francisco Veterans Affairs Healthcare System. He conducts applied research in positive health psychology with a special emphasis on self-forgiveness following perceived transgression. He has over 40 articles and chapters and an edited book to his credit.

M. Elizabeth Lewis Hall is a professor of psychology at Rosemead School of Psychology, Biola University. She has published widely on topics at the intersection of psychology and Christianity, including motherhood, sexism, self-objectification, embodiment, and meaning making.

Joshua N. Hook is an associate professor of psychology at the University of North Texas and studies positive psychology, humility, religion and spirituality, and multicultural counseling. He is the author of *Cultural Humility: Engaging Diverse Identities in Therapy* (2017) and *Helping Groups Heal: Leading Small Groups in the Process of Transformation* (2017).

Anthony Isacco is an associate professor of counseling psychology at Chatham University in Pittsburgh, Pennsylvania. His clinical practice is focused on the psychological assessment of Catholic deacons, seminarians, and religious women. He has published widely in the area of the psychology of men's health and has conducted specific empirical studies focused on Catholic priests and their health and well-being.

Sharon Y. Lee is a doctoral student in clinical psychology at the University of Connecticut. Ms. Lee studies the relationship between mental and physical health with respect to trauma and stress.

Gerdenio (Sonny) Manuel, S.J., is a professor of psychology, chair of psychology, and director of the Saint Ignatius Institute at the University of San Francisco. Fr. Manuel's areas of scholarship examine the relationship of psychology, faith, and spirituality in coping with stress and traumatic life events. He is the author of *Living Celibacy, Healthy Pathways for Priests* (2012).

Kate A. Meade is a doctoral student in counseling psychology at Chatham University in Pittsburgh, Pennsylvania. Her primary research interests are in the intersection of military trauma and sexual violence as well as the relationship between masculinity and sexual violence.

David M. Olson is a professor (physiologist) in the Department of Obstetrics and Gynaecology, Pediatrics and Physiology in the Faculty of Medicine and Dentistry at the University of Alberta. His research interests include parturition, preterm birth, and fetal development. His laboratory studies the various genetic, physiological, and environmental factors that contribute to both term and preterm labor.

Joanne K. Olson is a professor in the faculty of nursing at the University of Alberta. Her clinical area is community health nursing and health promotion. With past community health experience in rural, suburban, and urban settings in the United States and Canada, she continues to maintain a part-time clinical practice as a faith community (parish) nurse. Her research and scholarship has focused on nurse–client communication, spiritual aspects of nursing and health care, and nursing and interdisciplinary education.

Crystal L. Park is a professor of clinical psychology at the University of Connecticut. She has been conducting research on yoga for over eight years and recently developed, with colleagues, an NICCH-funded measure of the essential properties of yoga.

Luc R. Pelletier is a senior nursing specialist at Sharp Mesa Vista Hospital and adjunct professor, University of San Diego Hahn School of Nursing and Health Science, and health-care consultant in San Diego, California. His current research focuses on recruitment and retention strategies of new graduate nurses into the psychiatric–mental health nursing profession and the measurement of patient engagement in health care. He is the editor of *HQ Solutions: Resource for the Healthcare Quality Professional* (2018).

Ashley Pike is a social psychologist and a postdoctoral fellow in the Department of Occupational Therapy, Faculty of Rehabilitation Medicine, at the University of Alberta. Her clinical/academic career thus far has focused on scholarly, clinical, and academic contributions to mental health, offender rehabilitation, capacity building with correctional officers and health-care providers, building resilience, and implementation science. Presently, she is a research team member of a study funded to examine the health impacts of the 2016 Fort McMurray wildfires on pregnant women and their babies.

Kelsey Porada is a clinical research coordinator in Pediatrics at the Medical College of Wisconsin in Milwaukee, Wisconsin. She has published research on priest and seminarian well-being and has presented work at professional conferences.

T. Anne Richards is an interdisciplinary social scientist retired from the University of California San Francisco and Berkeley. She completed yoga teacher training at the 500-hour level at the Yoga Room in Berkeley. In 2013, Ms. Richards developed and piloted through the Public Health Institute a yoga program for women aimed at reducing incidence of urinary incontinence and associated distress. On a consulting basis, Ms. Richards assists in program development and evaluation at Curry Senior Center in the Tenderloin neighborhood of San Francisco.

Kalliope Sanderson is an undergraduate research assistant working with Crystal Park at the University of Connecticut. She is interested in the impact of mental health on well-being.

Shauna L. Shapiro is a professor at Santa Clara University and a clinical psychologist and specializes in mindfulness. She coauthored *The Art and Science of Mindfulness* (2009).

Timothy A. Sisemore has been in clinical practice for over 30 years and currently serves as a psychologist at Summit Counseling Center, Chattanooga, Tennessee. Among his articles and books is *Free from OCD, a Workbook for Teens with Obsessive-Compulsive Disorder* (2010) and the textbook *The Psychology of Religion and Spirituality: From the Inside Out* (2015).

Len Sperry is professor of mental health counseling and director of clinical training at Florida Atlantic University and clinical professor of psychiatry and behavioral medicine at the Medical College of Wisconsin. He is coeditor of the APA journal *Spirituality in Clinical Practice* and author of *Spirituality in Clinical Practice: Theory and Practice of Spiritually Oriented Psychotherapy* (2nd ed., 2011).

George Stoupas is an associate professor of human services in the addiction studies program at Palm Beach State College. He specializes in the addictions field, including the use of spiritual interventions to facilitate recovery.

Domenick Tirabassi is a doctoral student in clinical psychology at the Wisconsin School of Professional Psychology. His primary research interests are in the health and wellness of Catholic religious communities, priests, and seminarians.

Loren L. Toussaint is a professor of psychology at Luther College in Decorah, Iowa, and specializes in studying forgiveness and health. He has published over 80 articles and chapters as well as an edited book. He directs the Laboratory for the Investigation of Mind, Body, and Spirit.

Sandra Velasco-Scott has researched aspects of spiritual surrender of women with cancer participating in Psycho-Spiritual Integrative Therapy. Before earning her doctorate in psychology, she worked in church ministry for over 20 years and offers spiritual guidance in addition to various mental health interventions.

Sophie von Garnier is a graduate student in counseling psychology at Santa Clara University and researches positive emotions, mindfulness practices, and purpose in life. She graduated from Harvard University with a master of education in human development and psychology.

Amy Wachholtz is a clinical health psychologist, an assistant professor of psychology at the University of Colorado-Denver, and an assistant professor of psychiatry at the University of Massachusetts Medical School. Her research and clinical interests focus on the bio-psycho-social-spiritual model of pain disorders.

Kathleen Wall is a professor emerita in psychology at Sofia University, Palo-Alto, California and is a counselor/psychologist emerita from San Jose State University. She codeveloped Psycho-Spiritual Integrative Therapy and conducts research and trainings on it. This therapy integrates several psychotherapies, spiritual practices, and Integral Yoga philosophy.

Arielle Warner is a past research associate at Sophia University and has conducted cross-cultural research with Israeli, Palestinian, and American cancer survivors. She is on the faculty of Continuing Studies, Social Welfare and Health Sciences at Haifa University. She has a private practice in Israel focusing on spirituality and mental and physical health.

Everett L. Worthington Jr., is the Commonwealth Professor Emeritus in Psychology, Virginia Commonwealth University, and has published close to 40 books and over 400 articles and chapters in positive psychology and religion and spirituality.

Index